Safety-Wise

Girl Scouts of the U.S.A. 420 Fifth Avenue, New York, N.Y. 10018-2798

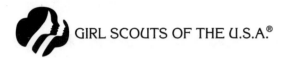
GIRL SCOUTS OF THE U.S.A.®

B. LaRae Orullian, *National President*
Mary Rose Main, *National Executive Director*

Inquiries regarding this book should be
addressed to *Safety-Wise*, Program Group,
Girl Scouts of the U.S.A., 420 Fifth Avenue,
New York, N.Y. 10018-2798.

Printed in the United States of America
First Impression 1993

10 9 8

Contents

Contents

How to Use This Book

Safety-Wise is addressed to all adults in Girl Scouting, with particular emphasis on those who work directly with girls.

This book has two objectives: to establish a safe and sound program experience that will protect and maintain the well-being of every Girl Scout, and to provide general safety guidelines as well as specifics for some common Girl Scout activities.

The chapter on "Girl Scout Program Standards" describes the essential components of a quality Girl Scout experience. The standards and their guidelines help adults to provide necessary health, safety, and security levels for girls. Every Girl Scout adult should be familiar with and adhere to each of the Girl Scout program standards.

The chapter on "Basic Safety and Security Guidelines" contains general guidelines that are fundamental to the prudent planning and smooth implementation of most Girl Scout functions.

The chapter on "Activity Checkpoints" provides a list of minimum requirements for common Girl Scout functions. Under typical Girl Scout activity headings, there are safety checkpoints for specific activities. They are to be used as extensions of the basic safety and security guidelines and Girl Scout program standards in the preceding chapters. For activities for which there are no checkpoints, the "Activity Considerations" section must be followed.

Additional activity checkpoints on caving, competitive orienteering, kayak-ing (sea and whitewater), playgrounds, ropes courses and rappelling, snowshoe-ing, and windsurfing can be found in *Safety and Risk Management in Girl Scouting*. These activity checkpoints are available through your local council.

The chapter on "Planning Trips with Girl Scouts" contains information on how leaders can work with girls to plan a variety of trips, including guidelines on preparation, evaluation, transportation, insurance, and a checklist for travel readiness.

The leader using this book for the first time should carefully read the Introduction, the chapter on "Basic Safety and Security Guidelines," and all the program standards. Once familiar with their content, you may look in the Table of Contents, the Index, or both for page references that apply to a specific activity the troop is planning. It will be important to also review the chapter on "Planning Trips with Girls." Terms important to health and safety in Girl Scouting are defined in the Glossary.

The leader must use *Safety-Wise* in conjunction with the leaders' guide for the age level with which she is working.

In all sections of *Safety-Wise*, the term "leader" is used for consistency and clarity of presentation. In interpreting the basic safety and security guidelines, activity checkpoints, program standards, and information about planning trips with girls, the term "leader" applies to the troop leader, assistant leader, leader-in-training, group coordinator, adult instructor of workshops or training sessions for girls, event or conference director, adult camp personnel, and program consultant.

The terms "troop" and "group" are also used for consistency. In interpreting the material in this book, leaders, program consultants, event and camp personnel, and other volunteer and employed council staff should recognize that these terms are used to describe gatherings of Girl Scouts in a variety of settings. The same safety and security guidelines, program standards, and activity checkpoints should be followed, whether traditional troop organization or any other form of grouping is used (for example, groups working on interest projects, service projects, or career activities, or participating in program events or activities in a camp, drop-in center, or program center). In addition, these safety guidelines, standards, and checkpoints apply equally to girls registered individually.

Throughout *Safety-Wise* the term "council" may be interpreted as "lone troop committee" for USA Girl Scouts Overseas.

All information used in preparing this publication is based on current nationally recognized materials available at the date of writing; therefore, councils need to keep abreast of changes.

Introduction

As Girl Scout program keeps pace with an everchanging world, health and safety remain cornerstones of the Girl Scout Movement. Sound health and safety principles must always permeate every Girl Scout activity. Safety should be planned, respected, and practiced by all. This does not necessarily imply burdens or restrictions. When Girl Scout members learn about safety, more activities are at their command. When safe practices are followed, participants can feel relaxed and confident. While one can never guarantee "total safety," it is possible to manage risk so as to reduce unnecessary risk.

In the United States, virtually every type of climate and terrain exists. As a result, different regions and councils have distinct and very different physical characteristics. To supply a set of comprehensive safety guidelines for every activity in every circumstance is impossible. Therefore, it should not be assumed that every single acceptable safety measure is contained in this publication or that additional measures may not be required. *Safety-Wise* offers general guidance that should be applied to specific situations. This guidance takes the form of Girl Scout program standards, basic safety and security guidelines, activity checkpoints, and advice on planning trips with Girl Scouts. The national organization provides this guidance for Girl Scout councils to use in supervising program activities carried out locally in troops, events, and camps. Through the council self-evaluation process GSUSA then monitors the council's ability to comply with GSUSA policies and standards related to health, safety, and security.

The Girl Scout Council

Each Girl Scout council is accountable for administering the delivery of Girl Scout program within its jurisdiction in a reasonably safe and secure environment. The council further provides direction for leaders through local guidelines, resources, and advice. In planning and guiding activities, councils establish local safety guidelines based on the standards and guidelines included in this book, *Safety and Risk Management in Girl Scouting*, and *Safety Management at Girl Scout Sites and Facilities*, as well as the council guides provided for individual resources at the different age levels. Each council must take into account local needs, geographic or climatic particulars, and state statutes and local ordinances that may be stricter than Girl Scout standards and guidelines.

In order to administer and implement a safe and sound Girl Scout program, the council must provide guidance and support to Girl Scout leaders by answering questions, providing training, suggesting resources, interpreting guidelines, selecting and approving sites, recommending program consultants for special activities, etc. All adult volunteers and employed staff should know the names, addresses, and phone numbers of the appropriate persons to contact in their Girl Scout council for guidance on safety and security issues. For USA Girl Scouts Overseas, the lone troop committee is the local authority responsible for these same accountabilities in consultation with the national organization.

The Girl Scout Troop or Group Leader

In Girl Scouting, the leader has the most contact with the girls, as well as the most impact on them. The examples the leader sets—of attitudes as well as actions—may well influence the lives of the girls.

In a sense, the leader, along with the parents, is responsible both for the girls and to the girls—for them, to safeguard their health; to them, to instill the sense of safe living that is so fundamental to their well-being. To accomplish these goals, all leaders must:

- Follow all the Girl Scout safety and security guidelines, program standards, and activity checkpoints.
- Follow all guidelines and procedures outlined by the council, including those that may supplement or augment GSUSA standards.
- Take appropriate training offered by the Girl Scout council.

- Use sound judgment in taking any additional precautions necessary to avert accidents.
- Be a role model. Set an example for health, safety, and security. (See the following guidelines.)
- Involve girls in safety planning and implementation.
- Nurture the concept of safety consciousness at all times, in all places.

But the leader is not expected to do all this alone. She should turn to the council for guidance and advice, and may also solicit the help of parents, program consultants, and other local resources. In addition, the girls participating in an activity should be expected to give cooperation and support.

Being a Health and Safety Role Model

Part of being an effective and responsible Girl Scout leader includes being a health and safety role model. Girls learn about health and safety directly and indirectly from the adults around them, and especially from their leaders.

The role of the leader in providing a healthy and safe Girl Scout environment is twofold: (1) the prevention of injury and illness to the individual while she is participating in a Girl Scout activity and (2) acting in a manner that shows concern for the health and welfare of the individuals for whom they are responsible.

Some examples of behaviors that show regard and respect for the health and welfare of girls and adults include:

■ Any kind of behavior that shows respect for local, state, and federal laws and ordinances.

■ Behavior that shows respect for the established policies of Girl Scouts as outlined in the *Blue Book of Basic Documents* and the *Leader's Digest*.

■ Behavior that shows respect for the standards, guidelines, and activity checkpoints set forth in *Safety-Wise* or those established by the council.

The following behaviors, which may threaten the health and welfare of girls, should be avoided when acting in an official Girl Scout capacity in the presence of girls:

■ Smoking. Research has shown the harmful effects of cigarette smoke to nonsmokers as well as smokers, especially children. Forgotten lit cigarettes have been known to cause fires.

■ Abuse of prescription, over-the-counter, or illegal drugs. Many readily available substances can be harmful if used incorrectly. Since many of these can be easily obtained by girls, it is very important for leaders to set an example.

■ Use of alcohol at girl activities. It is currently the most abused drug among youth in the United States. Alcohol and drug-related auto accidents are the leading cause of death among 15- to 24-year-olds.

Girl Scout councils may have their own policies that further outline a code of behavior to be followed when engaged in activities with girls and these are usually covered in basic leader training.

If you are unfamiliar with your council's policies or guidelines, contact your local Girl Scout council.

The Parent or Guardian

Parental involvement and support is an important ingredient in providing a positive experience for all girls in Girl Scouting. Each parent or guardian is urged to give assistance to the leader in ensuring the health, safety, and well-being of girls.

Each parent or guardian should:

■ Assist the leaders in planning and carrying out safe and secure program activities for girls.

■ Be willing to follow Girl Scout safety and security guidelines and standards and encourage her or his daughter/ward to do so also.

■ Participate in any parent/guardian meetings.

■ Give permission for her or his daughter/ward to participate in Girl Scouting and provide additional consent for activities that take place outside of the scheduled meeting place, involve travel, require the use of special equipment, or cover sensitive issues.

■ Make provisions for her or his daughter/ward to get to and from meeting places or other designated sites. Each parent or guardian should inform the leader of any changes in persons designated to drop off and pick up the child.

■ Provide her or his daughter/ward with appropriate clothing and equipment for activities planned, or contact the leader prior to the activity to find alternative sources for obtaining the necessary clothing and/or equipment.

■ Reinforce the concept of safety consciousness at home and in family activities.

The Girl

Girls who learn about and practice safe and healthy behaviors now will be better able to establish lifelong habits of safety consciousness. Each Girl Scout should:

■ Assist the leader in planning for safety.

■ Listen to and follow instructions and suggestions.

■ Learn and practice safety skills.

■ Learn to "Think Safety" at all times and to "Be Prepared."

■ Identify and evaluate situations where a safety risk is involved.

■ Know how, when, and where to get help when needed.

Every girl is an important link and every girl makes a difference.

Basic Safety and Security Guidelines

A positive attitude toward accident/incident prevention is the heart of safety and security consciousness. It involves a logical, natural way of anticipating risks and responding appropriately. For instance, on entering a car, buckling a seat belt becomes entirely automatic after doing it a few times.

Accidents and incidents are more likely to happen when safety and security precautions are overlooked. Mishaps usually don't occur when time is taken to plan ahead—when safe thinking lies at the base of all activities. For that reason, both adults and girls should strive to make safety part of their everyday thinking, to develop a safety/security consciousness.

Safety and security instruction, good supervision, and maintenance of safe surroundings can prevent accidents and incidents. Skill, good judgment, and quick action are also important aspects of safety and security.

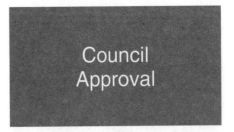

Good Judgment

Girl Scout leaders are always expected to exercise care and use good judgment. Judgment and common sense often dictate what is a safe and appropriate activity for girls. What is considered to be safe or appropriate in one set of circumstances might not be classified the same way in another set of circumstances. For example, weather conditions can change quickly and may call for good judgment in reassessing a situation and discontinuing an activity. When there is any question, the leader should provide the council with full details and not proceed without council approval.

The safety of the girls is the most important consideration. Children must be given a high degree of care. Because of their lack of experience and maturity, they need guidance and support from adults. Adults must determine the degree of care required, according to the age and skill of the child and the nature of the activity. It is better to err on the side of caution when considering whether to proceed with an activity.

Council Approval

Girl Scout leaders carry the responsibility for keeping the Girl Scout council and parents and guardians informed about the activities of the girls.

Any activity that may involve travel, cover subjects of a sensitive or controversial nature, or involve special equipment or supervision should be carefully considered and planned. It should be approved by the council and discussed with parents or guardians before it is included in troop plans. Remember, if there is a question as to whether a planned activity would fall into this category, the council should be consulted. It is the leader's responsibility to clearly describe the nature of the activity. Where the activity involves travel or special equipment, the leader should also outline all the preparation, training, and safety precautions that are planned.

In order to give its approval of a given activity, the council will need information about the "who, what, where, when, why, and how" of the activity. Program Standard 15 provides the detailed information that needs to be given to the council when seeking council approval.

Some specific activities, such as money-earning projects, certain types of service projects, and collaborations with other organizations, also require council approval.

Health Histories/ Health Examinations

As noted in the standard guidelines for Program Standard 3 (page 32), a health history is required annually for participation in physically demanding activities such as water sports, horseback riding, or skiing. A health examination within the preceding 24 months is required before a girl participates in resident camping, in a trip of more than three nights, or in sports on an organized competitive basis.

While obtaining health examinations may be financially difficult for some, they are necessary to protect the overall health and welfare of all the girls. For this reason, councils and leaders are urged to explore alternative means to meet this requirement. For example:

■ The health examination may be given by a qualified nurse practitioner, physician's assistant, or registered nurse working in cooperation with a licensed physician.

■ A girl may obtain a copy of her current school health examination record.

■ A girl may utilize community health services, such as the health department, the U.S. Army Medical Corps, and college or university medical schools.

■ The council may collaborate with an organization that is willing to sponsor a health examination clinic.

Clothing and Equipment

Girl Scouts participate in a variety of activities that take place in all types of climates and terrains. The appropriate clothing, supplies, tools, and other equipment will depend on the location and specific features of the activity. General suggestions are given, however, to help assist in the selection of proper clothing and equipment.

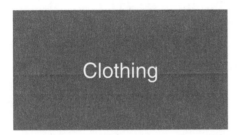

Clothing

Clothing and supplies should protect from environmental hazards such as sunburn, heatstroke, or hypothermia. In sunny, hot weather, sunblock creams and lotions and clothing covering shoulders and back will protect against painful sunburn. A protective lip balm will prevent chapped lips in all weather conditions.

The attire for an activity should also take into account such factors as poisonous snakes and plants, and bothersome insects and ticks. The weather forecast should be monitored as well as the nature of the terrain where the activity will take place.

Some general points to consider when advising girls on appropriate clothing are:

■ Uniforms provide identification for Girl Scouts traveling in groups.

■ Loose-fitting clothing allows for freedom of movement during strenuous activity.

■ Proper shoes and socks will be important to prevent fatigue, blisters, or general discomfort.

■ For warmth and partial protection against hypothermia, several light, loose layers of clothing insulate better than a bulky single layer of the same weight.

■ In the cold, a hat helps to retain body heat and in the heat protect against the sun.

■ Clothing made of wool insulates well even when wet.

■ Cotton will breathe and absorb moisture from the skin.

■ Dangling or flapping clothing can be a hazard, especially around playground equipment, machinery with moving parts, or around fires.

■ Clothing that is layered is the most effective means of meeting temperature changes. Waterproof gear should be used if there is a chance of getting wet, especially on cooler days when hypothermia becomes a real concern.

■ Clothing that covers arms and legs will provide protection from biting insects and ticks, poisonous plants, and sunburn; it also helps guard against bruises and scrapes in action sports (for example, roller skating, softball).

■ Sturdy boots with thick soles will protect feet on rugged, rocky terrain and help guard against bites from poisonous snakes.

■ Specialized clothing may be needed depending on the activity (for example, comfortable, sturdy shoes for hikes or extended walks; boots with heels for horseback riding; laced, tied, strapped on, or other nonslip footwear designed for water sports).

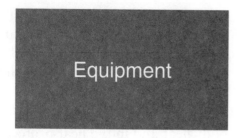

Equipment

Some general points to consider when advising girls on appropriate equipment use, care, and storage are:

■ The equipment should be appropriate for the activity.

■ Equipment should be suitable for girls with regard to age, size, maturity, experience, and ability. Girls should also use what is comfortable for them.

■ Rented or borrowed equipment, such as backpacks, skis, roller skates, and bicycles, should be selected, tested, and properly adjusted to accommodate each girl in terms of her size and ability.

■ Protective eye safety equipment, such as shatterproof lenses, eyeglass guards, or goggles should be worn when appropriate to prevent eye injuries in sports, arts and crafts, and science-related activities.

■ Appropriate protective devices, such as safety helmets, should be used in sports activities. Each type of safety helmet is designed to prevent injury for a particular activity. For example, bicycle safety helmets must be worn for bicycling. Horseback riding helmets must be worn for horseback riding.

■ Safety equipment (for example, belay lines, rescue bags, compasses, fire extinguishers, alarm equipment) should be used or be easily accessible and used when needed.

■ Equipment should be maintained in good condition. Equipment that appears defective should never be used. It should be repaired or disposed of. A safety check of equipment should be conducted prior to an activity.

■ Equipment that is regulated by legal standards must meet the specified requirements. For example, all personal flotation devices must be U.S. Coast Guard-approved and all horseback riding helmets must meet the American Society for Testing and Materials (ASTM) standards.

■ The manufacturer's instructions for safe use and care of equipment should be read and observed prior to putting any equipment into use. For easy referral, the manufacturer's instructions should be kept readily available and followed. All tools, equipment, and supplies (for example, power tools, poisons, paints, cleaning supplies, liquid fuels, and instruments with sharp edges) should be safely stored when not in use.

When girls are not properly equipped or clothed, they should not participate in the activity.

Preparation for the Weather

The enjoyment of any outdoor activity can be greatly affected by the weather. From basic comfort to general safety, it is always important to anticipate the potential weather conditions that may be faced and to be prepared. The following are some general guidelines:

■ In general, several layers of clothing are the best way to be prepared. A number of thin layers provide better protection against cold than one heavy layer. As the weather warms, layers can be removed.

■ Take precautions to prevent heat exhaustion. Loose, lightweight, and light-colored natural fiber clothing will help keep the body cool in hot weather. Drink plenty of water to prevent dehydration. Wear a lightweight head covering to protect the top of the head and shade the eyes. Be familiar with the following signs and symptoms of heat exhaustion:

▪ Cool and moist skin
▪ Heavy sweating
▪ Dilated pupils
▪ Headache
▪ Nausea
▪ Dizziness
▪ Vomiting
▪ Body temperature at or near normal

If you are alert for these signs you will be less likely to have to deal with heatstroke. On hot days, when the temperature is 80 ° F or above, and the activity calls for physical exertion, always be alert for the signs of heatstroke. Heatstroke is very serious and demands immediate medical attention.

■ Take precautions to prevent sunburn. Anyone can get a sunburn, even on a hazy day. Covering arms and legs helps, but burning rays can still penetrate light clothing to cause a sunburn. When using sunscreens or sunblocks, be wary about potential allergic reactions. Sunglasses, especially those that filter ultraviolet light, are also recommended. Remember that reflection from sand or snow increases the potential for sunburn.

■ Take precautions to prevent hypothermia in cool and cold weather. Waterproof clothing should be taken along if there is the potential for precipitation. Wet clothing, especially on a cool, windy day, can greatly increase the chance of hypothermia. The temperature doesn't have to be below freezing for this dangerous, potentially fatal, condition to occur. Be familiar with the following signs and symptoms of hypothermia:

▪ Shivering (may be absent in later stages)
▪ Dizziness
▪ Numbness
▪ Dilated pupils
▪ Apathy
▪ Loss of consciousness
▪ Decreasing pulse and breathing rate

Removing any wet clothing and rewarming the body gradually from the inside as well as outside are important first-aid steps. Seek medical assistance.

■ In freezing temperatures, be aware of the signs of frostbite. The skin usually turns chalky to grayish yellow in color and there is lack of feeling in the affected area. Warm the frostbitten area gently and don't rub. Seek medical help. If medical help is readily available or there is a possibility that the area may refreeze, avoid rewarming the affected area.

Preparation for Natural Disasters

Be prepared for the natural disasters that are most likely to occur in the region where an activity will take place. Here are some safety rules to follow for extreme weather hazards such as lightning, tornadoes, blizzards, flash floods, and hurricanes. Everyone should review and practice the procedures for seeking shelter and evacuating a site.

Lightning

Be very wary during thunderstorms. Lightning is responsible for many deaths each year. Lightning often strikes the tallest object in the area. At the first signs of an impending storm—towering thunderheads, darkening skies, lightning and thunder, and increasing wind—seek shelter.

If indoors, stay away from doors, windows, plumbing, and electrical appliances.

If caught outside during a lightning storm:

■ Don't seek shelter under tall, solitary objects, such as trees.

■ In open, flat areas, find the lowest point. Drop to a crouched knee position and bend forward, putting your hands on your knees.

■ Don't stand near any tall or metallic object.

■ Don't stand in or near any body of water.

■ Don't hold a radio, especially one with an antenna.

■ Don't hold an umbrella or any other metal object in an open area.

■ Seek safety inside a car.

Winter Storms

Winter storms vary in size and strength and may be blizzards, heavy snowstorms, or ice storms. When traveling during the winter, sufficient supplies of food, water, sleeping bags, and blankets should be taken to provide protection if stranded away from shelter.

The following precautions should be taken when caught in a winter storm:

■ Listen to a local radio station for a storm watch or warning. Have a battery-operated radio available in case of power failure.

■ Check battery-powered equipment, emergency cooking facilities, and other emergency gear.

■ Seek shelter and avoid traveling during a severe storm.

■ Conserve body heat and energy by avoiding overexertion from walking in the snow.

■ Use the buddy system when seeking help.

■ Know prevention and first-aid procedures for hypothermia and frostbite.

Floods and Flash Floods

Floods can occur almost anywhere and usually result from heavy or prolonged rain, rapidly melting snow, or dam breakage. Flash floods can occur with little or no warning and are dangerous because of their swift currents and unpredictable nature. The National Weather Service provides flood alerts. Radio broadcasts provide advance warnings and instructions.

When weather warnings are provided, evacuate the area swiftly and seek shelter. Extra food and water, flashlights, and dry clothes will be needed. If evacuation is not possible, determine the best route to high ground. Do not attempt to wade through water higher than knee-deep. Once high ground is reached, wait for rescue parties.

Hurricanes

The following safety rules should be considered before, during, and after a hurricane.

■ Listen for warnings on the radio. Have a battery-operated radio available in case of power failure.

■ Stay away from beaches or other locations that may be swept by tides or storm waves.

■ Watch for high water in areas where streams or rivers may flood after heavy rain.

■ If in a building with windows, board up all windows.

■ Store extra nonperishable food and water.

■ Make sure vehicles have gas.

■ Seek shelter indoors, away from windows.

■ Use the telephone only for emergencies.

■ Leave areas such as campsites that might be affected by the storm, tides, flooding, or falling trees.

■ Drive or walk to the nearest designated shelter, using recommended evacuation routes.

■ Do not be fooled by the "eye" of the storm (calm period). Winds from the other direction will soon pick up.

■ After the storm, stay away from disaster areas. Watch for dangling electrical wires, undermined roads, flooded low spots, or fires. Move cautiously.

Tornadoes

A tornado is considered one of nature's most violent storms because of its destructive force. Darkened skies, thick storm clouds, and strong winds from the south, combined with lightning and periods of rain and hail, often precede a tornado's arrival. If a tornado warning is issued, take a battery-powered radio and head for a protected area immediately.

Safe places to take shelter include:

- Storm shelters and basements

- Caves

- Tunnels and underground parking facilities

- Interior corridors or hallways

- Reinforced concrete buildings

Dangerous places that should be avoided include:

- Cars, house trailers, and parked vehicles

- Tents

- Structures with large, poorly supported roofs

- Gymnasiums or auditoriums

- Indoors near windows

If caught outside, move away at right angles to the tornado's path. If there is no time to escape, lie flat in a ditch, ravine, culvert, or under a bridge and protect your head.

Earthquakes

Earthquakes generally threaten areas along faults. The greatest danger from an earthquake is falling debris. Keep the following safety rules in mind when faced with an earthquake:

- Keep calm. Don't panic or run.

- If outdoors, get away from buildings, walls, utility poles, or power lines. Head for clear areas.

- If indoors, stand in a doorway or lie under a heavy piece of furniture such as a desk, table, or bed. Stay away from windows. Never run outside; you could be hit by falling debris or live wires.

- After an earthquake, don't enter buildings that have not been declared safe by authorities.

Emergency Procedures and First Aid

Emergencies can happen to anyone at any time and in any place. They require prompt action and quick judgment. First-aid treatment is essential within the first few minutes, because it can mean the difference between life and death. It is also vital to secure professional medical assistance as soon as possible.

Leaders are expected to see that girls receive proper instruction in how to take care of themselves and others in emergencies. To do this, leaders should help girls:

- Learn, plan, and practice how to administer emergency care in the event of simple accidents or of life-threatening situations.

- Become familiar with the safety measures outlined in their handbooks.

- Assemble a first-aid kit that is always accessible and stocked with necessary equipment (see list on pages 20 and 21).

- Understand and use the buddy system.

- Establish and practice fire evacuation, lost person, and security procedures.

- Know the three basic steps to take if clothing catches fire:

1. Stop.	Running only fans the fire.
2. Drop.	Lie flat.
3. Roll.	Rolling on the ground helps to smother flames. Or cover with a nonflammable material.

- Know what to report. Understand the importance of reporting accidents, illnesses, or unusual behavior to adults.

- Develop local emergency procedures that are written out, reviewed, and practiced.

First-Aid Courses

While first-aiders may not be required for regular troop meetings and activities not requiring physical exertion, they are needed for physically demanding activities or other activities involving a potential for injury.

The term "first-aider" is used throughout this publication. A Girl Scout first-aider is an adult who has taken Girl Scout council-approved first-aid training. All of these courses include CPR. There are two levels of first-aid care outlined for Girl Scouts.

Level I: The first-aid level is required for the adult acting as the primary first-aider for Girl Scout activities, programs, events, and overnight camping that meet two or more of the criteria for Level I first aid.

Level II: The second level is required for the adult acting as the first-aider in resident camp, core staff camp, family camp, events with more than 500 participants, trip camping of three or more nights, and camping events with over 200 participants or activities that meet three or more of the criteria for Level II first aid.

Leaders should take advantage of the first-aid training offered by local chapters of the American Red Cross, the National Safety Council, EMP America, or equivalent courses as approved by the Girl Scout council.

First-aid training is also recommended for girls. It is valuable in Girl Scouting, as well as in home and community life, and helps the girl expand her safety education. The American Red Cross, National Safety Council, EMP America, local rescue squads, and schools offer various safety training programs for young people.

Many other courses can increase the overall safety knowledge and skills of girls and adults. Courses in advanced first aid, swimming, basic water rescue, lifeguarding, and small craft safety can help ensure that an experience is the safest possible.

For further information on the training needed to become a first-aider and the criteria for each level, contact your council office.

First Aid and Infectious Diseases

Many first-aiders have expressed concerns about the possibility of contracting an infectious disease such as hepatitis B or the AIDS virus. To reduce the risks of becoming infected, the following precautions should be taken in all first-aid situations involving blood and other body fluids such as vomit, feces, or urine:

1. Gloves must be worn in every situation involving blood or other body fluids. Keep several pairs of latex gloves in all first-aid kits.

2. Cover open wounds with dressings to prevent the victim and first-aider from coming in contact with each other's blood.

3. Plastic wrap or other waterproof materials should be used to form a barrier if latex gloves are not available.

4. A pocket face mask or face shield with a one-way valve should be used when doing mouth-to-mouth resuscitation. This item should be in all first-aid kits.

5. After giving first aid, immediately wash hands and other skin surfaces coming in contact with body fluids thoroughly with disinfectant and/or antiseptic soap and water. Blood-soaked items or items that come in contact with body fluids should be placed in leakproof bags until they can be washed or disposed of. They should be washed in hot, soapy water. Clean reusable equipment and supplies first with detergent and water and then with a solution of one part chlorine bleach to ten parts of water. Rinse well. Gloves should be worn. **Note:** These procedures do not sterilize the equipment or supplies.

First-Aid Kits

A general first-aid kit should be available at the meeting place and accompany the girls for any activity, including transportation to and from an event. In addition to the standard materials, all first-aid kits should contain a copy of a recognized first-aid book, coins for telephone calls, and the Girl Scout council and emergency telephone numbers. Insurance forms, consent forms, and health histories should also be included. Prior to all activities, the kit should be checked to make sure that all material used previously or that may have expired has been replaced.

Whether you buy a commercially made kit or assemble your own, it should contain the following standard materials. In some instances, the purpose for the materials has been given to ensure that its use is clearly understood. The type, size, and contents of the kit will vary according to where it is to be used—for example, at the meeting place, or on a camping trip. Consult a physician for specific recommendations.

Adhesive tape and bandages

Alcohol wipes

Band-Aids, assorted

Bottle of distilled water (for use as an eye rinse or to clean wounds or other items)

Coins for phone calls

Flashlight

Gauze pads

Instant chemical icepack

Latex gloves (disposable for use in situations involving blood or other body fluids)

List of emergency phone numbers

Matches (for starting a fire)

Needle (for removal of splinters or to make small holes at the base of a blister)

Oral thermometer

Paper drinking cups

Plastic bags (for disposal of used materials and for collecting vomitus for analysis in suspected oral poisonings)

Pocket face mask or face shield (used in CPR for protection when performing mouth-to-mouth resuscitation)

Recognized first-aid book

Roller gauze bandages

Safety pins

Scissors

Soap (antibacterial liquid)

Splints

Triangular bandages

Tweezers

White index card, transparent tape, and self-closing plastic bag (for use when removing objects such as ticks. The item removed can be taped to the index card, enclosed in the plastic bag, and given to the medical professional.)

Additional supplies you may need: personal care products (for example, sanitary napkins or tampons).

Parents or guardians of any girls who are taking prescribed medications (for example, allergy pills) should inform adult leaders in advance. Any over-the-counter or prescribed medications should be in the original container and administered in the prescribed dosage by or in the presence of the responsible adult as per the written instruction by custodial parent or guardian or physician. Medication should never be given without prior written permission from a girl's custodial parent or guardian.

Council Procedures for Handling Serious Accidents, Major Emergencies, or Fatalities

It is important for each Girl Scout leader to observe council procedures for handling serious accidents, emergencies, or fatalities. Basically, at the scene of an accident, the adult in charge should first provide all possible care for the sick or injured. She should also follow preestablished council procedures for obtaining medical assistance and reporting the emergency. To do this, the leader must always have on hand the names and telephone numbers of the council representative, parents and guardians, and local emergency services such as the police, or a rescue squad. Many councils provide this information on a small card as a quick and easy reference.

After receiving the report, the council representative will immediately arrange for additional assistance (if needed) at the scene of the accident. She will also notify custodial parents or guardians and other appropriate persons.

In the event of a fatality or other serious accident, the police must be notified. A responsible person should remain at the scene. In the case of a fatality there should be no disturbance of the victim or surroundings until police have assumed authority. Information regarding the accident should not be shared with anyone but the police, the council's and volunteers' (if applicable) insurance representatives, and legal counsel.

Emergency Medical Care

As a result of an accident or injury, a minor may need emergency medical care. After contacting an emergency medical service, follow council procedures for incidents and accidents. Knowledge of and adherence to these procedures are critical, especially with regard to notification of a custodial parent(s) or guardian. In cases where the media are involved, the person designated by the council should be the only one to discuss the incident with these representatives.

Advance emergency release forms from the custodial parent(s)/guardian (granting permission for a minor's emergency medical care) should be obtained only through the council. The council should not solicit advance emergency release forms from custodial parent(s)/ guardian (granting permission for a minor's emergency medical care) without first investigating the laws in the community where the Girl Scout activities are to take place. This step will ensure that such forms are valid there.

The council should also have statements available for use by parents who object to their daughter receiving medical care for religious reasons.

Fire Evacuation Procedures

The leader, with the assistance of the girls, should design a fire evacuation plan for meeting places used by the group. If a school or other public building is used, follow the plan that has been established for that facility once you have made certain that it will work during the time the group is there. Every girl must know where to go and how to act in case of fire. The following points should be considered in designing a fire evacuation plan:

- Draw a floor plan showing all exits and potential escape routes.

- Determine more than one way out in case an escape exit is blocked.

- Designate a meeting place outside.

- Locate a fire alarm box or accessible telephone outside the meeting place.

- Review the plan with the girls.

- Practice the plan with a representative from the local fire department.

- Request that the plan be posted in a conspicuous place.

- Conduct fire drills periodically.

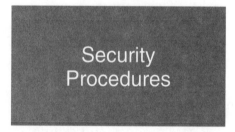

Security Procedures

The leader, with the assistance of the girls, should develop a security plan for the meeting place or activity area. This plan should include procedures for determining the number of girls and their whereabouts at all times. Head counts should be conducted before and after every activity. It should also include measures to help ensure that the site is safe. Every girl must know where to go and how to act when confronted by strangers or intruders and be able to sound an agreed-upon alarm.

Local Emergency and Disaster Procedures

Girl Scouting occurs in many different climates and terrains with potential emergency conditions. In anticipating such emergencies, the Girl Scout council should assist leaders in planning local emergency procedures. When advance warnings of impending emergencies are issued, activities already planned for that area must be canceled. If an activity is already in progress, appropriate measures must be taken to safeguard the girls. To do this, plans for shelter and evacuation from the meeting place, campgrounds, and all other sites should be known to all, posted, and practiced in advance.

Local emergency management or civil defense departments, the disaster committees of Red Cross chapters, safety councils, weather bureaus, park systems, state or U.S. Forest Service, and the Army Corps of Engineers may provide assistance to leaders, girls, and councils in developing appropriate procedures for their locale.

When troops or groups are engaged in activities beyond their own locale, it is important to learn about potential emergencies and disasters in the places to be visited.

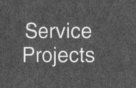

Service Projects

Girls may not participate in service projects that involve health and safety risks—for example, service projects requiring specialized training or certification, such as lead paint removal.

Service projects involving litter pick-ups, stream cleanup, adopt-a-highway programs, and other such activities that involve girls, adults, and/or families picking up trash to beautify an area, need to be carefully planned because they present the following risks:

- Unless all debris is disposed of properly and completely, the Girl Scout council involved with the cleanup may be held liable for its illegal disposal.

- Having children clean up along highways being used by fast-moving vehicles can present the possibility of a serious accident, unless careful coordination is established with the highway patrol or local police.

- There can be a serious disease potential involved in having children pick up trash, which may consist of discarded drug needles, medical wastes, etc.

Guidelines
for Sensitive
Issues

In order to remain contemporary and responsive to the needs and interests of girls, some of the activities in Girl Scout program focus on subjects that may be considered sensitive or controversial in nature. There is not a definitive list of these subjects. In general, topics that are of a highly personal nature, such as human sexuality, or that may relate to religious beliefs and cultural and family values, should be regarded as sensitive. Subjects such as AIDS, child abuse, suicide, and teenage pregnancy are examples. A certain amount of judgment is required since what may be considered sensitive in one part of the country or to one group of people might not be classified the same way in another section of the country or for another group. Many subjects have the potential to become controversial if handled inappropriately. Therefore, it is important to know and follow any council procedures for handling sensitive issues.

When Girl Scout program activities focus on or include sensitive or controversial issues, the role of the leader is to be a caring adult who can help girls acquire their own skills and knowledge in a supportive atmosphere rather than one who presents any particular position of advocacy.

The Issues for Girl Scout series does not contain information or activities that are any more sensitive or controversial than what is currently printed in Girl Scout handbooks for each age level. While leaders should have acquired skills in facilitating program activities and girl planning before introducing these materials, they are not required to have specific training for each topic covered in Issues for Girl Scouts. However, when implementing these resources, adults need to be sensitive to the particular values and practices in their communities.

Since most sensitive topics are rooted in values, parental support and understanding are crucial to the success of all activities on these topics. Involving parents and guardians in the activities that girls do in a troop or group meeting or at home would go far toward reassuring them of the quality and benefits of these activities. (See Program Standard 10 on "Parental Permission.") When deciding to cover any sensitive issue beyond the scope of the materials in the Girl Scout program resources, the leader must have the support and approval of the council.

In many cases, program consultants and special resource consultants are utilized to deliver program on sensitive issues. They should understand and be willing to adhere to Girl Scout national policies and the Girl Scout position on human sexuality and other related topics.

When discussing value-related topics, the leader should encourage girls to talk with resource people, such as family members, religious leaders, and experts in a particular field. It is important for a girl to hear all sides of a question and to be guided by her own parents and the teachings of her religious group before she tries to make a decision. Girls should be encouraged to see that each family has its own way of doing things based on family customs, religion, cultural background, lifestyles, and so on. Girls should also be encouraged to try to understand parental decisions by examining the parent's point of view.

The leader should help girls to consider the possible consequences of an action they are considering. Girls need to see the importance of weighing future implications of an action against the immediate result.

Girl Scouting plays a vital role in helping girls to make informed, responsible decisions about their well-being. The leader should assure girls of her trust in them and her confidence in their ability to make decisions that are correct for them.

Tips for Handling Specific Sensitive Issues

If a Girl Scout leader notices signs of substance abuse, child abuse, suicide, eating disorders (anorexia nervosa and bulimia), she should notify her council or follow council procedures that may have been established. If the leader does not feel comfortable reporting this information directly, there should be an adult whom she trusts that she can report it to. That person can then take appropriate action. Reporting information to people who can help is the most vital step in protecting children. In some cases, it is also the law.

The following are some general tips for how to handle specific sensitive issues. More detailed information is included in the Contemporary Issues or Issues for Girl Scouts booklets for the topic discussed.

Substance Abuse

Many young people are abusing one or more substances and many more are being pressured to do so. Alcohol is the most socially acceptable drug in our society and is the most abused drug among youth in the United States, followed by tobacco.

The following are possible signs of drug involvement. Keep in mind that these signs can also be attributed to other stresses in a girl's life.

■Abandonment of goals and reduction of ambitions

■Withdrawal from school and family activities

■A drop in quality of schoolwork and in grades

■Increased secretiveness

■Changes in friendships

■Changes in behavior—including disruptive, delinquent behavior

■Erratic mood changes, apathy, and lethargy

■Disappearance of money and other valuables

■Neglect of personal appearance and hygiene

■Presence of drug paraphernalia, incense, room deodorizer, eyedrop bottles, drugs

■Chronic lying

- Physical symptoms such as red eyes, sores on nose or mouth, fatigue, drowsiness, loss or gain in appetite, altered speech, puncture marks on arm

- Sudden constant runny nose

- Eating extremes, unexplained weight loss

- Dulled speech and expression

- Wearing sunglasses unnecessarily

- Avoidance of eye contact

- Changes in speech patterns, including slang terms, profanity

- Overreacting, overly sensitive responses

- Problems with concentration and memory

If you notice these signs, follow the guidelines of the council for reporting this information.

Child Abuse

Child abuse affects over 1.5 million children each year in the U.S. Physical abuse, sexual abuse, emotional maltreatment, and physical neglect are the four common types of abuse.

Most abused children show some of the following symptoms: low self-esteem; anger; guilt; aggressive, hyperactive, or disruptive behavior; withdrawal; delinquent behavior; poor school performance; and abuse of drugs and alcohol. More than one of these symptoms is usually present in cases of child abuse. The Contemporary Issues booklet *Staying Safe: Preventing Child Abuse* contains more specific signs for each type of abuse.

Since child abuse is a crime, an agency in every state is mandated by state law to receive and to investigate reports of suspected child abuse. In some states, Girl Scout leaders are considered to be mandated reporters. The leader should check with her local Girl Scout council to determine her responsibilities for reporting.

If a girl tells you she has been abused, the following should be done:

- Treat what the girl has said as fact

- Assure her it is not her fault and that it is important that she told someone about it

- Be sympathetic and nonjudgmental

- Consult with your council contact to determine appropriate next steps

Some symptoms that may signal a girl is in an abusive situation or has been abused are:

- Unexplained injuries such as bruises, burns, or fractures

- Excessive fearfulness or distrust of adults

- Abusive behavior towards other children, especially younger ones

- Avoidance of physical contact

If you suspect a girl has been abused but she has not specifically told you about it, the following should be done:

- Consult with your council to determine the appropriate course of action

- Report the suspected abuse to the agency in your state mandated to receive and investigate such cases

Since abuse can happen in any environment, it is important that volunteers and staff who work directly with girls do the following:

■Be familiar with and observe all council guidelines related to preventing child abuse

■Follow adult supervision guidelines outlined in this book and any additional guidelines that the council has established to assure that there is no risk of any abusive situation within the Girl Scout setting

Suicide

Every year in the United States, more than five thousand young people commit suicide and as many as a half million more attempt to do so. Suicide is the third-leading cause of death among adolescents.

Any suicide threat should be taken seriously. Talk to a reliable family member or guardian. Appropriate council personnel and/or health care professionals should be notified.

An essential part of suicide prevention lies in being alert to the warning signs of suicide. These are some of the specific signs that indicate that a girl might be a suicide risk:

■Long-standing depression (sometimes manifested as boredom, agitation, acting-out behavior, or physical symptoms such as headaches). The times when a girl is going into and apparently recovering from depression are particular danger points.

■Eating and sleeping disturbances

■Declining academic performance and/or inability to concentrate

■Previous suicide attempts, suicidal gestures, or verbal suicidal

threats or other statements indicating a desire to die

■Withdrawal from family and friends

■Fatigue, apathy, or loss of interest in activities that were previously enjoyed

■Marked changes in behavior or personality (for example, unusual moodiness, aggressiveness, or sensitivity)

■Deterioration in appearance and personal hygiene

■Giving away prized possessions

■Preoccupation with the subject of death

■Recent traumatic events, such as the death of a family member

■Feelings of worthlessness and hopelessness, of not being loved or appreciated

If a girl seems to be suicidal or has made a suicidal threat:

■Don't pull away from her. Remember that suicidal adolescents rarely seek out professional help on their own.

■Trust your instincts. Don't ignore the warning signs.

■Don't offer reassurances that may not be true.

■Offer to help her, but don't agree to keep information confidential if she reveals something that might affect her safety.

■Be sympathetic.

■Reassure her that she does have someone to turn to and that she can be treated.

- Contact your council contact to determine appropriate action.

- Don't leave her alone if the situation is immediately life-threatening. Call a responsible family member or even the police, if necessary.

Eating Disorders

Anorexia nervosa and bulimia are eating disorders characterized by a preoccupation with food, an irrational fear of being fat, and a distorted body image. Anorexia involves a dramatic weight loss due to self-starvation or severe self-imposed dieting. Bulimia involves binge eating and purging accompanied by frequent weight fluctuations, rather than extreme continuous weight loss. It is estimated that anorexia strikes more than one in every one hundred teenage girls and young women; the rate is much higher for bulimia.

If a girl is suspected to be bulimic or anorexic, try to talk with her about the problem. Since these disorders can be serious, at times even life-threatening, early detection and treatment are crucial. Alert parents or guardians, and contact the council office for sources of professional help. The friendships found in Girl Scouting can be an important adjunct to therapy, and should be supported.

AIDS

AIDS stands for Acquired Immune Deficiency Syndrome, a disease in which the body's immune system breaks down. AIDS is caused by the virus called human immunodeficiency virus or HIV. It is important to know how the virus is, and is not, spread.

The AIDS virus can be spread through sexual contact with an infected person, sharing unsterilized needles or syringes that have been used by an infected person, through blood transfusions prior to 1985, and during pregnancy if the mother is infected. AIDS is not spread by sneezing, coughing, or by touching doorknobs, toilets, dishes, clothing, or other things in the home or outside the home.

Since there is a risk of infection when blood and other body fluids are involved, girls and adults should take the necessary precautions outlined on page 20.

Situations may arise when leaders suspect a girl is HIV positive or has AIDS. It is important to follow council procedures for handling such situations. To date, it has been determined that children testing positive for the AIDS virus do not pose a risk to others in a school or social setting. None of the cases of AIDS in the U.S. are suspected to have been transmitted from one child to another in the home, at school, at foster care, or in a day-care setting. On the contrary, the child whose immune system is damaged by AIDS is highly susceptible to infections from other children in a school or social setting. Assessment of risk from participation in Girl Scout troop/group activities can most accurately be made by the child's physician.

Remember, knowing what to do in advance will help you to respond effectively to situations involving sensitive issues.

Girl Scout Program Standards

The Girl Scout program is an informal educational program designed to help girls put into practice the fundamental principles of the Girl Scout Movement as set forth in the Preamble. It is carried out in small groups with adult leadership and provides a wide range of activities developed around the interests and needs of girls.

—*Constitution of Girl Scouts of the United States of America,* Article III

The 35 program standards provide a means for determining a desired level of performance and for meeting the basic levels of health, safety, and security that must be provided to girls.

Every Girl Scout adult who is involved with girls, either directly or indirectly, should be familiar with each of those standards. Individually they specify the necessary elements of a quality program experience. Collectively they ensure that all Girl Scouts will benefit from a rewarding educational experience carried out in a way that safeguards the health, safety, and general well-being of all involved.

Each standard is followed by a set of guidelines. These statements further describe each standard, providing examples and details to more fully illustrate what must be done in order to meet the standard.

The standards are organized under five major subsets: Girl Scout Program, Adult Leadership Roles and Responsibilities, Troop/Group Management, Transportation, and Money Earning/Troop Financing.

Standards 1 and 2 set out basic requisites that apply throughout all the other standards. For example, activities are based on the needs and interests of girls and their overall readiness. This applies whether it is an outdoor, money-earning, or service activity.

Some standards require greater amplification than others, but this does not mean that any standard is more important than another. When specific information in one standard draws upon important information in other standards, those standards are listed in the guidelines. In other instances, the guidelines will refer you to another section of the book. It is most important to follow these directions, since they will provide you with critical information related to the standard. You will also find references to other Girl Scout resources that contain additional information related to the standard.

Girl Scout Program

1

Girl Scout Program—Foundation and Goals

Program experiences and activities should meet the needs and interests of girls, be based on the Girl Scout Promise and Law, and enable girls to grow and develop, as described in the four Girl Scout program goals.

Standard Guidelines

A The Girl Scout program has four fundamental goals, and the experiences and activities enable each girl to:

1 Develop to her full individual potential.

- Foster feelings of self-acceptance and unique self-worth.
- Promote her perception as competent, responsible, and open to new experiences and challenges.
- Offer opportunities to learn new skills.
- Encourage personal growth.
- Allow girls to utilize and practice talents and abilities.

2 To relate to others with increasing understanding, skill, and respect.

- Help each girl develop sensitivity to others and respect for their needs, feelings, and rights.
- Promote an understanding and appreciation of individual, cultural, religious, and racial differences.
- Foster the ability to build friendships and working relationships.

3 Develop values to guide her actions and to provide the foundation for sound decision-making.

- Help her develop a meaningful set of values and ethics that will guide her actions.
- Foster an ability to make decisions that are consistent with her values and that reflect respect for the rights and needs of others.
- Empower her to act upon her values and convictions.
- Encourage her to reexamine her ideals as she matures.

4 To contribute to the improvement of society through the use of her abilities and leadership skills, working in cooperation with others.

- Help her develop concern for the well-being of her community and its people.
- Promote an understanding of how the quality of community life affects her own life and the whole of society.
- Encourage her to use her skills to work with others for the benefit of all.

B The four program goals provide direction for Girl Scout program that is adapted to meet the developmental, educational, emotional, and social needs and interests of girls at five age levels.

Applicable membership standards are as follows:

- Daisy Girl Scout (K–grade 1 or 5–6 years old)
- Brownie Girl Scout (grade 1–3 or 6–8 years old)
- Junior Girl Scout (grade 3–6 or 8–11 years old)
- Cadette Girl Scout (grade 6–9 or 11–14 years old)
- Senior Girl Scout (grade 9–12 or 14–17 years old)

C Girls with mental retardation should be registered as closely as possible to their chronological age. They wear the uniform of that age level. Adaptations should be made of the ongoing activities of the age level to which the troop belongs. Young women who are mentally retarded may retain their girl membership through their twenty-first year and then move into an adult membership category.

2

General Activities

Program activities should include a balance of subject and interest areas. The types of activities should be determined in partnership by the girls and their leaders and reflect the girls' needs and interests, physical and emotional readiness, skill level, and preparation. The activities should provide for progressive learning experiences, both at the current age level and in preparation for the next one.

Standard Guidelines

A Activities include opportunities for:
- Cooperative learning experiences
- Experiential learning
- Individual and group participation
- Value development
- Decision-making
- Skill building
- Exploration of roles and contributions of women past, present, and future

■Respect for and understanding and appreciation of cultural, religious, ethnic, and racial diversity

B Activities should be varied in type and subject matter. The Girl Scout worlds of interest provide a general reference for a wide range of topics.

C Activities should be planned with sensitivity to varying needs and abilities of girls in language skills, proficiency in English, and mental and physical disabilities.

D The handbooks, recognition books, and other supplemental resources are used to plan and guide the activities.

E For additional guidance on specific activities, see the "Activity Checkpoints" chapter.

F Ceremonies are held to emphasize important moments in Girl Scouting, including:
■Investiture
■Rededication
■Court of Awards
■Fly-up and Bridging
■Thinking Day
■Girl Scouts' Own

(*Ceremonies in Girl Scouting* and the various handbooks provide further information on these and other ceremonies.)

3

Health, Safety, and Security— Activity Planning and Implementation

At all times, the health, safety, and security of girls should be paramount. All activities should be planned and carried out so as to safeguard the health, safety, and general well-being of girls and adults. Girls and adults should follow proper safety practices at all times.

Standard Guidelines

A In planning an activity with the troop/group, the leader should note the abilities of each girl and carefully consider the progression of skills required to go from the easiest part of the activity to the most difficult. She should make sure that the complexity of the activity does not exceed the girls' individual skill levels, bearing in mind that skill levels will decline when the participants are tired, hungry, or under stress.

B Girls and leaders should learn and follow health and safety practices as outlined in this text and in each of the basic Girl Scout program resources.

C In any group, an effective level of discipline should be maintained so that needless risks are avoided.

D A health history (see Glossary) and an activity permission form (see Appendix) signed by the parent or guardian are obtained before a girl participates in physically demanding activities. Information in a health history is confidential.

E A record of health examination (see Glossary) given by a licensed physician, a qualified nurse practitioner, a physician's assistant, or a registered nurse under a physician's orders within the preceding 24 months is required before a girl participates in resident camping, in a trip of more than three nights, or in contact sports on an organized competitive basis. Information from a health examination is confidential and should only be shared with persons who have a need to know in order to protect the health and safety of the participant and other participants. If there is a religious reason for not having such an examination, there is a signed statement by a religious leader to that effect. The statement may include accommodations that are determined to be necessary to allow participation in the activity. If the leader cannot determine how the accommodation(s) may be accomplished, she should ask the council for assistance.

F Anyone who has a known complicating medical problem, or who has had a serious illness or injury or an operation since her last health examination, submits a written statement from her physician or religious authority, if her religion precludes the use of a physician, giving permission to participate in any activity that normally requires a current health history or health examination.

4

International

Girl Scouting is part of a worldwide movement, and program activities should emphasize this international dimension.

Standard Guidelines

A Girls understand the significance of the World pin and the meaning of WAGGGS, the World Association of Girl Guides and Girl Scouts.

B Program activities for girls promote multicultural understanding and appreciation of diversity—geographic, economic, racial, ethnic, religious, etc.

C Girls are familiar with the activities and recognitions in their handbooks, recognitions books, etc., that inform them about the international scope of the Girl Scout/Girl Guide Movement.

D Girls learn about their responsibilities and potential to contribute to a global society.

5
Service

Service is inherent in the Promise and Law and is given without expectation of payment or reward. All girls should take part in service activities or projects.

Standard Guidelines

A Service activities or projects are determined by the girls and the needs of the community.

B Councils provide support to girls in identifying potential service projects, locating resources, and planning service projects.

C Awards are not provided for hours of service. However, girls may be recognized for special training, skill development, leadership, and accomplishments, and some form of

written documentation indicating the service rendered may be given to girls for their records.

6
Experiences Beyond the Troop/Group

Girls should have experiences that broaden their perspectives and enable them to interact with individuals beyond their immediate group. Program activities should provide girls with opportunities to have experiences beyond regular troop/ group meetings.

Standard Guidelines

A When activities take place outside the scheduled meeting place, parents and guardians should be informed and asked to provide written consent. See Standard 10, pages 36–37.

B Refer to the "Planning Trips with Girl Scouts" chapter for further amplification of this standard.

C Girls should have the opportunity to interact with other troops at the same and at different age levels.

7

Outdoor Education

Activities carried out in outdoor settings are an important part of Girl Scout program for each age level. The leader should receive the appropriate training from her council to help her guide preparation for and implementation of the outdoor activities.

Standard Guidelines

A All activities in an outdoor setting reflect an understanding of the importance of conserving and improving the environment and protecting wildlife.

B Prior to their activities, girls learn about and practice skills they will use.

C *Outdoor Education in Girl Scouting,* the audiovisual *From Backyard to Backcountry: Camping Lightly on the Land, Earth Matters,* and *Exploring Wildlife Communities with Children* provide information and guidance for outdoor-related activities.

8

Girl Scout Camping

Girl Scout camping should provide girls with a fun and educational group living experience that links Girl Scout program with the natural surroundings and contributes to each camper's mental, physical, social, and spiritual growth.

Standard Guidelines

A Leaders receive council training before taking girls troop camping.

B Girls and their leaders work with the Girl Scout council in planning a Girl Scout camping experience. See Standards 6, 13, 14, 18, 22, 23, 24, 25, 26 and activity checkpoints for Troop Camping.

C Girls and adults prepare for the camping experience.

D Girls learn about and practice minimal-impact camping. (See the audiovisual *From Backyard to Backcountry: Camping Lightly on the Land.*)

9

Girl Scout Recognitions

Girl Scout recognitions should acknowledge a girl's accomplishments and attainment of specified requirements. Leaders should work in partnership with girls to decide when recognitions, such as badges, patches, or awards, have been completed. At all times, adults should play a key role in stressing the quality of the program experience over quantity of recognitions.

Standard Guidelines

A The selection of recognitions is based on the girl's interests, with leader guidance, and is not leader-directed.

B Leaders help girls understand the purpose of each recognition.

C Leaders assist girls in planning activities to complete recognitions.

D Program activities are not structured solely to fulfill recognition requirements. Leaders help girls appreciate the fun and value of doing something for its own sake, not just to obtain a recognition.

E Credit is given for continuity of membership and for badges and activities, when properly recorded, to girls who have been affiliated with other troops or groups or with recognized organizations within the World Association of Girl Guides and Girl Scouts.

10

Parental Permission

Written permission from a parent or legal guardian should be obtained for participation in Girl Scouting. Leaders and girls are responsible for informing parents or guardians of the purpose of Girl Scouting; of the date, time, and place of meetings; and of the type of activities included in troop plans. When activities take place outside of the scheduled meeting place, involve travel, or focus on sensitive or controversial topics, parents and guardians should be informed and asked to provide additional written consent.

Standard Guidelines

A Leaders inform parents or guardians about proposed activities outside of the scheduled meeting place that involve travel or that cover sensitive or controversial issues, and discuss such activities with them before plans are developed.

B Leaders consult with council representatives before undertaking any activities involving special equipment or supervision, or sensitive or controversial issues. See pages 56–59 for further information.

C Leaders obtain a parent's or guardian's written permission for every girl wishing to participate in an activity, or a series of activities, that is held at a different place and time from the regularly scheduled meeting place and time, or that involves unusual risks or controversial issues.

D Leaders seek assistance in ensuring that a lack of proficiency in English is not a barrier to parental participation and input.

E Permission forms are developed with council guidance. (See suggested form on page 142.)

11
Girl Scout Membership Pins and Uniforms

All Girl Scout members should wear the membership pin when participating in Girl Scout activities. Since Girl Scouting is a uniformed organization, girl and adult members should be informed, at the time they become members, that they are entitled to wear the Girl Scout uniform appropriate for their age level. Although the wearing of the uniform is encouraged, it should be clearly conveyed that the wearing of the uniform is not required for participation in Girl Scouting.

Standard Guidelines

A Members who do not own uniforms wear the Girl Scout membership pin appropriate for their age level.

B Uniforms are not required for members to participate in Girl Scout activities.

C Girl Scout uniforms can be an important contributor to group identity and promote a greater sense of unity and parity among members at each age level.

D Guidelines for wearing the uniform appropriately are followed. (*Girl Scout Uniforms, Insignia, and Recognitions* and the various handbooks contain specific details.)

E When appropriate, the official uniform is used to identify traveling troops and groups or individuals representing the organization.

12

Girl/Adult Partnership

Girls and their leaders should work as partners in planning and decision-making. Tasks should be sensitive to girls' developmental maturity and commensurate with their abilities, with each girl encouraged to proceed at her own pace. With each age level, the girls' opportunity to act independently and handle responsibilities should increase.

Standard Guidelines

A Simple forms of government, as outlined in the girls' handbooks, are used to promote leadership skill development.

B With each age level, the degree of guidance by the adult leadership is matched to the age and maturity of girls. Daisy Girl Scouts depend largely on leader direction, while Senior Girl Scouts plan with maximum independence.

C Leaders are sensitive to the varying needs and abilities of girls, including those related to language skills and to physical and mental disabilities, to ensure that every girl may participate fully.

D Leaders, program consultants, or outside instructors working with girls have the skills, competencies, and preparation required for the type of activity and its level of difficulty.

E Leaders assist girls in:
- Learning decision-making skills
- Assuming a variety of responsibilities
- Selecting activities that match abilities and encourage growth
- Proceeding at their own pace
- Understanding and accepting that learning experiences involve both successes and failure

Adult Leadership Roles and Responsibilities

13

Troops/Groups

Each troop or group should have at least one adult leader and one or more assistant leaders. Because the female role model is essential to fulfilling the purpose of Girl Scouting, at least one member of the leadership team must be an adult female.

The adult leaders must be at least 18 years of age or at the age of majority defined by the state if it is older than 18. Leaders should have training as specified by the council. In addition, an active troop committee of registered adult members should provide ongoing support to the troop.

Standard Guidelines

A During all troop meetings and in all related small-group activities, there should be present the leader, the assistant leader, or other responsible adult designated by the leader or by the council, and at least one of these must be an adult female.

B Recommended ratios of adults to girls are:

For meetings—

■ Two adults to every:

　10 Daisy Girl Scouts
　20 Brownie Girl Scouts
　25 Junior Girl Scouts
　25 Cadette Girl Scouts
　30 Senior Girl Scouts

■ Plus one adult to each additional:

　　5 Daisy Girl Scouts
　　8 Brownie Girl Scouts
　10 Junior Girl Scouts
　12 Cadette Girl Scouts
　15 Senior Girl Scouts

For events, trips, and troop camping—

■ Two adults to every:

　　5 Daisy Girl Scouts*
　12 Brownie Girl Scouts
　16 Junior Girl Scouts
　20 Cadette Girl Scouts
　24 Senior Girl Scouts

■ Plus one adult to each additional:

　　3 Daisy Girl Scouts*
　　6 Brownie Girl Scouts
　　8 Junior Girl Scouts
　10 Cadette Girl Scouts
　12 Senior Girl Scouts

*Under the leadership of the troop leader, and with parents, guardians, or other family members, a Daisy Girl Scout troop may participate in occasional overnight family camping experiences.

C The troop leadership team helps to recruit three to six members for the troop committee and keeps them informed about the troop plans. The troop committee members are registered Girl Scout adults who provide the principal support to the leader, supplying transportation, assistance with projects, leader substitutes, etc.

D A member of the troop's sponsoring group is on the troop committee. This committee serves as a communications link between the sponsor and the troop.

E Girl Scouts who are leaders-in-training (LIT) and counselors-in-training (CIT) may supplement the regular adult leadership required but are not substitutes for adults.

F Any adult volunteer whose behavior is not in keeping with the standards set forth in this book, as well as those established by the council, may be asked to relinquish her or his position.

14

Health, Safety, and Security— Adult Supervision and Preparation

Proper adult supervision and guidance for each activity are essential. Adults with requisite expertise are part of the adult leadership when implementing activities. Adequate training and preparation for girls and adults precede participation in any activity.

Standard Guidelines

A When preparing for any activity, general health and safety considerations are reviewed (see pages 11–28).

B The "Activity Checkpoints" chapter of this book is consulted for specific information. When a contemplated activity is not included in the activity checkpoints, a council representative, program consultants, advisers, and qualified personnel are contacted to provide direction and guidance, and to grant approval as required.

C When an activity is planned on a topic of a sensitive or controversial nature, parents and the council are informed and permission is received before proceeding.

D When any activity is planned in which special equipment, training, or expertise is required, the council is consulted to ensure proper approval, supervision, and insurance coverage.

15

Council Support to Adult Leadership

All adults within the Girl Scout council work in concert to ensure the highest quality program experience for girls. Communication and cooperation are essential for providing training, giving ongoing support to troops and groups, and obtaining appropriate activity approvals.

Standard Guidelines

A Troop leaders and assistant leaders take advantage of basic and advanced program training and other adult education opportunities pro- vided by the council or by council-approved outside organizations.

B The Girl Scout leader is responsible for obtaining council permission for trips and special activities and keeping the council informed of ongoing troop/group activities.

C The leader provides the following information to the council when seeking approval for a given activity:

- Identity of the troop or group involved
- Location and type of activity
- Type of premises
- Inclusive dates and times
- Number and ages of girls participating and parental permissions obtained
- Number of adults participating, their gender, and in what capacities
- Skill level of the participants
- Safety precautions planned
- Special consultants or resource people who will be involved
- Other groups or organizations involved
- Specialized equipment being used
- Itinerary
- Mode of transportation
- Specific activities involved
- Any special agreements or contracts required (for example, hiring a bus, use of premises)

16

Program Consultants

The regular adult leader-ship of any Girl Scout group should be complemented by program consultants who possess technical competence and the ability to share specialized skills.

Standard Guidelines

A Program consultants are recruited to provide enrichment activities and share specialized skills. They should:

- Possess technical competence
- Be willing to follow Girl Scout program goals and practices
- Be willing to cooperate with the leader in carrying out the project
- Be able to be an appropriate role model for girls

B The leader briefs the consultant on:

- Girl Scout program standards (for example, basic program goals)
- Basic safety and security guidelines
- Girls and their abilities, as well as ongoing troop plans

17

Program Centers

All centers and facilities used for Girl Scout program activities should have present at least one adult with appropriate qualifications and competencies to guide girls in the type of program conducted at the facility. Additional adults trained for their particular roles should be present in numbers required to provide adequate adult guidance for the ages of the girls, the size of the group, and the nature of the activity.

Standard Guideline

A The average ratios of girls to adults in a program center are two adults (**at least one of whom is female**) to every:

10 Daisy Girl Scouts
20 Brownie Girl Scouts
25 Junior Girl Scouts
25 Cadette Girl Scouts
30 Senior Girl Scouts

■ Plus one adult for each additional:

5 Daisy Girl Scouts
8 Brownie Girl Scouts
10 Junior Girl Scouts
12 Cadette Girl Scouts
15 Senior Girl Scouts

18

Adult Leadership— Girl Scout Camps

All Girl Scout camps should be staffed by adults who possess the qualifications and necessary competencies for the positions held.

Standard Guidelines

A Each and all groups of participants will be led by adults, at least one of whom is an adult female.

B See Standards 14, 15, and 22.

Troop/Group Management

19

Pluralism and Diversity of Troops/Groups

Girl Scout troops and groups should reflect the diversity of socioeconomic, racial, ethnic, cultural, religious, and disability groups in the community. Whenever possible, troops and groups should include girls from different age and grade levels.

Standard Guidelines

A Leaders and girls respect the beliefs and practices of all religious, ethnic, racial, linguistic, and socioeconomic groups in the troop/group membership.

B In choosing meeting places, selecting meeting dates and times, planning activities, considering schedules for trips, making group menus, etc., consideration is given to the needs, resources, safety and security practices, and beliefs of all members, and to the special needs of any members who have disabilities.

C The selection of the troop committee and program consultants reflects the diversity of the community.

D See Standard 1 for guidelines related to serving girls with mental retardation.

20
Size of Troops/Groups

Girls should be able to participate in groupings large enough to provide experience in self-government and in groupings small enough to allow for development of the individual girl.

Standard Guidelines

A With the exception of Daisy Girl Scout troops, girls should meet in groups that permit interaction with individuals from more than one school grade.

B Ratios of girls to adults provide appropriate adult leadership (see the Guidelines for Standard 13).

C It is recommended that the troop and group sizes be as follows:

Daisy Girl Scouts	5–15 Girls
Brownie Girl Scouts	15–25 Girls
Junior Girl Scouts	15–30 Girls
Cadette Girl Scouts	10–30 Girls
Senior Girl Scouts	10–30 Girls

21
Meeting and Activity Planning

Troops and groups should meet often enough to fulfill the needs and interests of girls and to maintain continuity of their program experience.

Standard Guidelines

A The schedule of the meetings and other activities is worked out by the girls in partnership with the leaders or other adults who work with them.

B To permit full participation, factors such as school schedules, family needs, scheduled events, religious holidays, safety concerns, and availability of transportation and meeting places are considered when planning meeting times.

22

Meeting Places/Camps/Sites

All meeting places, camps, and other sites used for Girl Scout program activities should provide a safe, clean, and secure environment and allow for participation of all girls.

Standard Guidelines

A All places selected for activities are easily accessible to all members, including girls with disabilities.

B The meeting area meets the following criteria:

- It is safe, secure, clean, properly ventilated, heated, lit, free from obvious hazards, and has at least two exits.

- The area is large enough for a variety of activities.

- First-aid equipment is on hand.

- It has accessible toilets and sanitary facilities.

- It is accessible to telephones or other communication equipment.

- Emergency exits are functioning, easily accessible, adequate, and well marked.

- If the activity will extend into dusk, adequate lighting is present.

23

Girl Scout Camps

All Girl Scout camps should be operated in compliance with local and state laws for maximum protection of campers' health, safety, and security, and with regard to protection of the natural environment.

Standard Guidelines

A Girl training includes skill development and health and safety procedures that will enable them to be cooperative participants at camp and derive maximum benefits from the experience.

B Arrangements to attend Girl Scout camp are completed according to council procedures.

24

Overnight Trips, Camping

All sites and facilities used for overnight trips or camping should be approved by the Girl Scout council.

Standard Guidelines

A It is the leader's responsibility to inform the council of any planned trips and to obtain needed permissions.

B See Standards 3, 6, 8, 13, 14, and 15.

Transportation

25

Private Transportation

Private passenger cars, station wagons, and vans may be used during Girl Scout activities. They must be properly registered, insured, and operated by adults with a valid license for the type and size of vehicle used. Any other form of private transportation may be used only after council approval has been obtained.

Standard Guidelines

A The number of passengers does not exceed the intended passenger limits of the vehicle. Each person has her or his own seat and uses a seat belt.

B There is adequate space for luggage and equipment, which is stowed securely.

C Vehicles are used for their intended purpose. Trucks and similar vehicles used to transport equipment and supplies are not used to transport anyone in the area designed for cargo. Trailers or other towed vehicles are not used to transport passengers. Exception: Vehicles designed for hauling and in good condition may be used for hayrides on private property or for floats in parades. (For further information, see pages 134–137.)

D Vehicles designed primarily to serve as recreational homes are used to transport only the number of persons for which there are specifically designed passenger seats.

E All vehicles should be equipped with a first-aid kit and any federal- or state-required safety equipment (for example, spare tire, reflective devices, fire extinguishers, personal flotation devices).

F The section on transportation on pages 134–137 of this book should be consulted for further information about arranging transportation.

26

Public Transportation

Public transportation and regularly scheduled airlines, buses, trains, and vessels should be used whenever possible.

Standard Guideline

A See Guidelines B, E, and F under Program Standard 25.

27

Travel Procedures

All travel procedures and preparations should make provision for adequate adult supervision and maximum safety.

Standard Guidelines

A Group transportation procedures drawn up by the local council, in accordance with local regulations, are followed.

B All girls have received training, and all safety rules and procedures are reviewed prior to the trip.

C Adequate adult supervision is provided (see Program Standard 13).

D All passengers are considerate of the driver and observe all safe conduct rules for the form of transportation used.

E Adequate rest periods are provided for drivers. A rest stop should be scheduled at least every two hours.

F Precautions are taken to avoid fatigue of passengers.

G There are prearranged meeting places if two or more vehicles are involved. Caravaning (convoy-type travel) is avoided because of the dangers inherent in trying to stay together on a busy highway and the potential hazard of collision.

H All passengers receive instructions in emergency procedures (for example, how to evacuate a bus, how to signal for help from the roadside or on the water).

I A trip plan is left with a designated person at the council office.

J In planning any trip, the leader follows all applicable recommendations in the chapter "Planning Trips with Girl Scouts."

Money Earning/Troop Financing

28

Activities Involving Money

Troops/groups should be financed by troop/group dues, by troop money-earning activities, and by a share of money earned through council-sponsored product sales. Daisy Girl Scouts may not be involved in handling any money, including troop dues and proceeds from troop money-earning activities and product sales.

Standard Guidelines

A "Troop money earning" refers to activities planned and carried out by girls and adults, in partnership, to earn money for the troop treasury, following a planned budget.

B "Council-sponsored product sales" are councilwide sales of authorized products, such as Girl Scout cookies or calendars, in which troops participate.

C Girls at all age levels except the Daisy Girl Scout level engage in troop budgeting activities that help them to learn money management. The girls are part of the decision-making process in determining troop dues, troop money-earning projects, and uses of collective funds. The funds are for Girl Scout activities and are not to be retained by individuals as their property.

D Daisy Girl Scouts are not involved in handling any money, including troop dues. Adults associated with the Daisy Girl Scout troop—leaders, parents, etc.—handle money and meet the modest cost of the troop's activities.

E Permission is obtained in writing from a girl's parent or guardian before she participates in troop money-earning projects or council-sponsored product sales.

F Girls' participation in troop money-earning projects or council-sponsored product sales is based on the following:

■ Voluntary participation

■ An understanding and ability to interpret to others why the money is needed

■ Correct business procedures

■ Observance of local ordinances related to involvement of children in money-making activities

■ Adherence to guidelines for personal protection

■ Advance provision for safeguarding the money

G Girl Scouts may not earn money for other organizations. However, girls may contribute a portion of their troop treasury to organizations or projects they consider worthwhile (for example, local or international community-service organizations or environmental projects).

H Girls should be encouraged to designate a portion of their troop treasury for the annual membership dues of all troop members. This is a sound and efficient practice that enables girls to meet membership dues and lessens the potential burden to individual members.

I See activity checkpoints for Cookie/Council-Sponsored Product Sales.

J See also Program Standards 29, 30, 31, 32, and 33.

29

Troop Money-Earning Activities

Money-earning activities should be a valuable program activity for girls. Daisy Girl Scouts do not participate in troop money-earning activities.

Standard Guidelines

A Troop leaders obtain written approval from their council before starting a troop money-earning project.

B The number of money-earning projects does not exceed what is needed to support troop activities, and the amount to be raised is determined in accordance with a previously prepared troop budget.

C Troop money-earning activities are suitable to the ages and abilities of the girls and are consistent with the goals and principles of Girl Scout program. Some examples include making items and selling them; washing cars; putting on plays or puppet shows, etc. Games of chance, direct solicitation for cash, or endorsement of a commercial product are not appropriate money-earning activities.

D The experience gives girls the opportunity to learn multiple skills, such as budgeting, goal setting, customer relations, good business practices, and public relations.

E When girls participate in money-earning activities outside their troop meeting place, an adult is present at all times. Parental/guardian permission is obtained.

F The troop submits a complete report on the troop money-earning activities, including evaluation, to the council.

G In no case does the income from troop money-earning activities become the property of individual girl members.

30

Council-Sponsored Product Sales

Troops/groups may participate in no more than two council-sponsored product sales each year, and only one of these may be a cookie sale. A percentage of the money earned through product sales should be allocated to participating troops and groups. Daisy Girl Scouts may not sell cookies or other products.

Standard Guidelines

A The selling of Girl Scout cookies or other council-sponsored products is a valuable program experience for girls. This activity should not be assumed by adults. Refer to activity checkpoints for Cookie/Council-Sponsored Product Sales.

B Parents and guardians grant permission and are informed about the girls' whereabouts when they are engaged in product sales.

C Brownie Girl Scouts should have an adult present. Junior Girl Scouts should have an adult present or they may be teamed with a Senior Girl Scout. Girls should work with other Girl Scouts and be identifiable as Girl Scouts by wearing a membership pin or uniform or carrying a membership card. The buddy system must be practiced.

D Money for products sold is collected when the products are delivered.

E Girl members who participate in Girl Scouting through alternative membership patterns, rather than a troop, are allowed to participate in council-sponsored product sales. In such instances, the total proceeds resulting from their efforts are retained by the council to provide program activities and mailings for those members who are not affiliated with a troop.

F In no case does the income from product sales become the property of individual girl members.

G The percentage of money to be allocated to participating troops is determined by the council and interpreted to leaders prior to the product sale.

31
Product Sale Incentives

Participation in a council product sale incentive plan should be optional for troops and individuals. Incentives, if used, should be program-related and of a type that will provide opportunities for girls to participate in Girl Scout activities.

Standard Guidelines

A Examples of suitable incentives are camperships, event fees, day camp fees, scholarships for wider opportunities, and materials and supplies for program activities.

B If the council has an incentive plan, the plan should apply equally to girls in troops and to those participating in Girl Scouting through alternative patterns of membership.

32
Council Fund Raising

Fund raising or fund development to support the Girl Scout council is the responsibility of adults and this responsibility should not be placed with girls. Girls may provide support to these efforts through voluntary service.

Standard Guidelines

A "Fund raising" or "fund development" refers to any of various methods of soliciting contributed funds—for example, annual campaign, capital campaign, project funding, planned giving, benefits, and federated funds allocation.

B Some examples of suitable ways for girls to support the council's fund-raising efforts include speaking about Girl Scout program, stuffing envelopes for an annual fund-raising campaign, assisting at a fund-raising function by carrying out a flag ceremony, escorting dignitaries, putting together a slide show, etc.

33

Fund Raising for Other Organizations

Girl Scouts, in their Girl Scout capacities, may not solicit money for other organizations. Girl members may support other organizations only through service projects. (See national policy on solicitation of contributions in the Leader's Digest: Blue Book of Basic Documents.*)*

Standard Guideline

A Some examples of suitable service projects to support other organizations include stuffing envelopes, delivering informational pamphlets to businesses, helping to organize and catalog books for a library book sale, serving as aides, or providing record-keeping assistance.

34

Collaborations with Other Organizations

When collaborative relationships or cooperative projects are developed with other organizations, all Girl Scout program standards are followed.

Standard Guidelines

A Cooperative relationships are established only with organizations that have goals and practices compatible with Girl Scouting.

B Council approval is obtained for cooperative projects.

C The organization representatives are briefed on all Girl Scout program standards, policies, and practices.

35

Political Activity

Girl Scouts, in their Girl Scout capacities, may not participate directly or indirectly in any political campaigns or participate in partisan efforts on behalf of or in opposition to a candidate for public office.

Standard Guidelines

A   Girl Scouts are encouraged to become active and knowledgeable citizens, but must maintain a nonpartisan stand when acting in an official Girl Scout capacity. Wearing the uniform, citing a troop number or council affiliation, or otherwise identifying oneself as a Girl Scout are examples of when one is acting in an official Girl Scout capacity.

B   Girl Scouts may express their opinions and beliefs when acting as individual citizens.

C   Letter-writing campaigns, circulating petitions, or carrying banners or signs at political rallies and functions are all examples of partisan political activity.

D   See the policy on political and legislative activity in the *Blue Book of Basic Documents.*

Activity Checkpoints

The checkpoints in this chapter give quick guidance for the planning and implementation of specific activities. The checkpoints represent the basic minimums to follow. Because of the many different sites and circumstances surrounding any Girl Scout event, these checkpoints are not all-inclusive. The checkpoints may serve as starting points for investigating resources with more in-depth information. When local conditions raise questions about interpretation of any of the guidelines, consult with your council. The council can assist in implementation of an activity that meets the intent of the guidelines and address considerations specific to a particular area.

Supervision

A certified instructor or adult who has documented experience in a particular activity is required for most aquatic activities and certain activities that demand specialized skills, equipment, and supervision. The following list provides some guidance on how to develop proper documentation for equivalent training/experience and competence of leadership:

- Course requirements that match those specifically listed in *Safety-Wise*
- Performance reviews from prior employers, mentors, and/or the council
- Prior work experience, including dates and job descriptions
- Results of training/testing/review provided by certified staff with proper documentation
- Grades in appropriate courses (with course contents attached)
- References from people with documentation indicating that they are competent to make a statement about the applicant's competence
- Certified translations of certificates/references in languages not understood by the supervisor

Before beginning any activity, the leader or responsible adult must:

- Be familiar with all of the program standards and related guidelines.
- Review the activity checkpoints.
- Obtain the written permission from parents or guardians if necessary.
- Obtain council permission, if necessary.

■ Refer to the Girl Scouts of the U.S.A. program resources for guidance. The handbooks for girls, leaders' guides, and other supplemental resources outline activities carefully designed to bring the best possible experiences to girls.

Aquatic Supervision Ratios

When planning aquatic activities, a safety network for all girls and adults is of primary importance. The safety network is a shared responsibility. Each girl or adult who participates in aquatic activities must be accountable for her own behavior by conducting herself according to the rules of the waterfront, including following instructions, swimming in assigned areas, watching out for her buddy, etc.

Aquatic activities must be carefully supervised by instructors or leaders who have current certification and/or documented experience in specialty areas such as swimming, windsurfing, or whitewater kayaking.

The number of persons who supervise a given aquatic activity is determined by the skill level of the swimmers, degree of risk, and environmental conditions. Council guidance must be obtained in determining the acceptable procedures for conducting any swimming or boating activities.

Swimming

Swimming Activities in pools, lakes, slow-moving streams, and rivers:

Lifeguard-Watcher Ratio Chart		
Number of Swimmers	Lifeguards	Watchers
1–10	1+	1*
11–25	1+	2*
26–35	2+*	3*
36–50	2+*	4*

+ Primary lifeguard must be an adult.

* May be a person who is under the age of majority for the state in which the activity will take place, but cannot be under 16 years of age.

Note: At no time can the number of lifeguards and watchers under the age of majority be greater than the number of adult lifeguards and watchers. For swimming in backyard pools, use one lifeguard for 1–10 swimmers. The lifeguard must be a minimum of 16 years old, with certification in American Red Cross Lifeguard Training or equivalent. An adult trained in water rescue skills must also be present.

Swimming Activities in oceans, large bays, or wide, rapidly running rivers:

One currently certified adult lifeguard for every 10 swimmers, plus one watcher.

The ratio of lifeguards and watchers to swimmers may need to be increased depending upon the following factors:

■ Number of girls in one area

■ Swimming level and ability

■ Girls with disabilities (depending on the types)

- Age level and ability to follow instructions
- Type of swimming activity—instruction, recreation
- Type of swimming area
- Weather and water conditions
- Types of available rescue equipment

Boating

- For every boating activity, a minimum of two qualified adults must be present.
- One adult must be a certified instructor/qualified leader for the type of craft.
- One adult must be certified in American Red Cross Small Craft Safety or have documented training and experience in river rescue or the equivalent, as appropriate to the type of craft and aquatic environment.

Specific instructor/qualified leader to participant ratios have been established for boating activities that involve greater risk and require more stringent supervision. Those ratios are written under the checkpoints for the activity.

The leader to participant ratios for boating activities may be increased, depending upon a variety of factors:

- Number of craft
- Size of craft
- Age level of girls
- Number of girls and craft
- Experience level of girls

- Type of activity—instruction, recreation, tripping, etc.
- Difficulty of activity
- Size of body of water
- Wind conditions
- Tides and currents
- Flatwater or whitewater
- Turbidity
- Bottom conditions
- Shoreline
- Other boats in proximity

Activity Considerations

When a troop wants to plan an activity, the checklist that follows will help determine whether it is appropriate to do so. This list should be used especially when considering an activity that is not described in this book.

- Is the activity educationally sound?
- Will the activity contribute to fulfilling each of the program goals stated after Program Standard 1?
- Is knowledgeable, trained, experienced leadership available?
- What resources are required, including financial resources, equipment, instruction, etc.?
- What potential health and safety risks are involved?

■ Have parents/guardians been advised through parental permission forms of potential health and safety risks, special equipment needed, and/or required skills or experience?

■ Are the girls physically, emotionally, and intellectually ready?

■ Is the activity a logical progression in skill building?

■ What are the possible risks and how will they be handled?

■ What are the overall benefits of the experience for the girls?

■ What impact will there be on the environment?

■ Is the site selected appropriate for the activity?

■ Is council permission required?

■ Is parental permission required?

Some activities are demanding physically, emotionally, and in terms of skills. Many such activities offer challenging experiences that may promote girls' growth and development, but may also involve a wide range of variables that require extensive planning and expertise to control. With activities that require specialized skills, training, and equipment, care must be taken to control risks as much as possible, ensure that participants are prepared for the activity, and make sure the activity is conducted under optimum safety conditions. Extensive consideration must be given to any decision to undertake these activities. The skill and training required of participants and leader/facilitators must be carefully assessed and monitored.

Because of unpredictable variables, certain activities can carry risk even when they are conducted with extreme skill and care. **The following are not permitted as Girl Scout program activities:**

■ High altitude climbing

■ Hang gliding

■ Bungee jumping

■ Ballooning

■ Flying in small private planes, helicopters, sailplanes, and blimps

■ Paintball

■ Parachuting

■ Parasailing

■ Trampolining

■ Hot dog skiing

■ Riding motor bikes

■ Riding in all-terrain vehicles

■ Go-carting

■ Using personal watercraft (a small motor-driven craft that may be ridden in a sitting position like a snowmobile or standing as in skiing)

■ Watercraft trips in Class V and above whitewater

If there are any other questions about the appropriateness of any activity, the leader or responsible adult should contact the council for further guidance.

When permission is received to conduct an activity not described in this chapter, the following list should be used to write specific checkpoints for the activity.

Health History and Health Examination

A health history and/or health examination may be necessary, depending upon the type and duration of the activity.

Planning and Supervision

■ Instructors with certification from a recognized organization or equivalent certification, or with documented experience in the activity, must be selected.

■ The instructors must meet any state or national qualification/certification requirements that may exist.

■ A girl's participation depends on her readiness: her level of maturity, physical conditioning, and level of training. A girl must not be pushed beyond her capabilities.

■ Girls must be instructed in basic and advanced skills as necessary.

■ Instruction must be adequate and with proper progression.

■ Safety rules must be reviewed and practiced.

■ The ratio of adult supervisors to girls must be adequate for the degree of risk and level of skill involved in the activity.

■ The activity must be evaluated by all involved.

Clothing and Equipment

■ All equipment must be appropriate for the activity.

■ All equipment must be in good working order and properly adjusted for each participant.

■ Girls must wear protective clothing appropriate for the activity and the weather.

■ Safety equipment appropriate for the activity must be used and be easily accessible, such as ropes, throw bags, fire extinguishers, etc.

■ Rented or borrowed equipment must be carefully inspected before use by someone familiar with such equipment for obvious hazards. Instruction books must be read before equipment is needed.

Transportation

■ If transportation is needed before, during, or after the activity, arrangements must be made in advance.

■ Plans must be confirmed before departure.

Site

■ Council guidance and approval must be obtained in selecting a site.

■ The facility must be appropriate for the skills and ability levels of the girls.

■ The safety rules related to the specific activity must be written, posted, understood, and practiced by all.

■ Respect for the environment must be demonstrated.

■ Weather conditions must be suitable and monitored.

Emergency Procedures and First Aid

■ An adult with current first-aid training must be present.

- First-aid equipment and supplies appropriate to the activity must be available.

- First-aid procedures appropriate to the activity must be understood and practiced.

- Emergency medical care must be accessible.

- Accident/incident report forms must be available and used if needed.

- The itinerary must be left with a contact person at home. The contact person must be called upon departure and return.

- A list of emergency telephone numbers must be written and posted.

- Specialized safety and rescue procedures appropriate to the activity must be understood and reviewed, including procedures that involve team effort.

- Security plans and procedures must be established prior to activity participation.

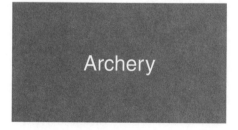

Archery

Archery is not recommended for Daisy or Brownie Girl Scouts. A participant in archery activities must be old enough to understand safety procedures and handle equipment with proper caution toward other participants and onlookers.

Planning and Supervision

☐ One adult must be a currently certified National Archery Association Instructor or have equivalent certification or documented experience indicating knowledge and skill in teaching/supervising archery.

☐ Instructors must have thorough knowledge of safety practices, equipment use and maintenance, and technique.

☐ A ratio of 1–10 participants to one instructor must be observed.

☐ Rules and operating procedures must be reviewed with the girls prior to each session.

☐ The safety rules must be written, understood, practiced, and posted at the shooting site.

☐ A system for alerting participants about starting, retrieving, and emergency stopping must be in effect.

☐ Girls must develop skills based on proper procedures and form, such as bow stringing, nocking the arrow, stance, sighting, and observing safety practices.

For both outdoor and indoor archery ranges:

☐ Archers must straddle the shooting line to shoot.

☐ Girls waiting to shoot must be behind the shooters.

☐ A ground quiver for arrows must be provided for each line of shooters.

❏ Rules must be written, understood, practiced, and posted.

❏ Any archery games undertaken away from a regular course must be well supervised and must be appropriate to age, skill level, and location of shooting.

Equipment

❏ Bows and arrows must be appropriate to the age, size, strength, and ability of the girls.

❏ Girls must have finger and arm protection such as finger tabs and arm guards. Right- and left-handed models must be made available.

❏ All equipment must be checked prior to use.

❏ Arrows must not be warped or have cracked nocks or loose or missing feathers.

❏ Bowstrings must not have broken or loose strands.

❏ Bows must not have loose or broken arrow rests.

❏ Backstops for targets must be in good repair.

❏ Arrows for a beginner must be long enough to extend one to two inches in front of the bow when a girl has the bow at full draw. Use target tip arrows only, **never** broadhead tips.

Transportation

❏ Provision must be made for safe handling of archery equipment to and from the range.

Site

❏ All equipment must be secured in a dry, locked storage area.

Additional Checkpoints for an Outdoor Range

Safety considerations must dictate where an outdoor range site will be located. Targets must not be placed in front of houses, roads, trails, or tents. Avoid areas that have any pedestrian traffic. Clear areas of brush. A hillside backstop is preferable.

❏ The shooting area and spectator area behind the shooting area must be clearly marked.

❏ The shooting area must include a distance of at least 50 yards behind the targets and 20 yards on each side of the range.

❏ An outdoor range must not be used after nightfall unless there is proper lighting to maintain the safety of participants.

Additional Checkpoints for an Indoor Range

❏ An indoor range shooting distance must be a maximum of 20 yards.

❏ Targets must be well lighted.

❏ Any doors or entries onto the range must be locked or blocked from the inside. (Do not block fire exits.)

Emergency Procedures and First Aid

❏ An adult with current first-aid training must be present.

❏ A first-aid kit must be available.

❏ In the event of an electrical storm, seek low ground and shelter. If a sheltered area is not available, crouch low to the ground in an open area. Do not stand under tall, solitary objects such as trees or electrical poles.

❏ A written safety plan must be in use.

National Organizations

American Archery Council, National Archery Association.

Arts and Crafts

Planning and Supervision

❏ With younger age levels, age-appropriate materials and tools must be used. For example, always use water-based paints and products that are easily removed from clothes. Scissors must have a blunt end.

❏ For activities that extend beyond those described in the Girl Scout handbooks and other related materials, the instructor must have documented experience indicating knowledge and skill in teaching arts and crafts.

❏ The instructor must teach girls the basic skills and demonstrate the safe use and care of equipment—for example, cutting tools must be used with the blade away from the body; girls must never mold a paintbrush tip with their lips, etc.

❏ Activities must be appropriate in terms of each girl's experience in working with tools, her age and attention span, and the complexity of the project.

❏ Cutting tools, hammers, and spray paints require close inspection prior to use and careful instruction in their use.

❏ Kilns must be ventilated, and children must not use them without direct supervision.

❏ Supervision must be increased when advanced equipment, such as soldering irons, burners, or power saws, is used.

❏ Girls must wash their hands after using potentially toxic supplies.

Clothing

☐ Girls must wear appropriate protective clothing. This may include gloves for handling hot objects and masks or goggles for protection against sparks, dust, fumes, or debris.

☐ Long hair must be tied back, and loose clothing and jewelry must not be worn when using machinery or tools with moving parts.

Equipment and Materials

☐ Equipment and supplies must be ample for each group.

On November 18, 1988, the U.S. Congress passed Public Law 100-695, The Labeling of Hazardous Art Materials Act, requiring that all chronically hazardous art materials carry a statement that such materials are inappropriate for children and that the Consumer Product Safety Commission may bring legal action to forbid the purchase of chronically hazardous art materials for use by children in grades six and below. Art materials manufactured and labeled since October 1990 are mandated to include chronic hazard warnings where needed.

The Arts and Crafts Materials Institute (ACMI) has developed and instituted a voluntary program that attempts to provide standards for the safety of childrens' art materials. Products that bear their labels are marked—AP (Approved Product) and CP (Certified Product).

Choose products whose labels clearly indicate what the material is and how to write or call the manufacturer. Purchases of art materials should be made from reputable sources, such as school supply houses.

Caution must be taken to protect children from dyes, pigments, preservatives, and other chemicals that may provoke allergies. Children who are physically or psychologically disabled, or who are on medication, may be at greater risk from toxic materials. **The following materials may be used after girls have received adequate safety instruction:**

☐ Dusts or powders that can be inhaled or that can get in the eyes.

☐ Organic solvents, volatile glues, or solvent-containing products, such as aerosol spray cans.

☐ Anything that stains the skin or clothing (or that cannot be washed out of clothing).

☐ Acids, alkalis, bleaches, or other irritating or corrosive chemicals.

Girls should never use:

☐ Any donated or discarded material for which the ingredients are not known, or very old or unlabeled materials that may be toxic.

The following are some safety points for the handling and storage of equipment and supplies:

☐ Equipment and supplies must be locked in a storage area whenever possible.

☐ Safety and operating instructions for potentially dangerous equipment (for example, power tools, kilns) must be reviewed and posted.

❑ Scissors, knives, and other cutting tools must be kept clean, oiled, and sharpened, as needed.

❑ Flammable materials, such as paints and solvents, must be labeled and stored in a dry, well-ventilated area out of the reach of young children.

❑ Equipment and supplies must be used for their intended purpose only.

❑ Turpentine or paint thinner may be used as a paint solvent with adequate ventilation. Gasoline must never be used as a paint solvent.

❑ Solvent- or oil-soaked rags must be kept in waste cans that meet fire safety codes and are emptied daily.

❑ Solvents must be covered. They evaporate quickly, and inhalation can be hazardous.

❑ When using natural materials to be gathered by girls, care must be taken to teach and practice conservation principles.

❑ Manufacturers' labels on paints, chemicals, and aerosol cans must be read before use. These substances must always be used in well-ventilated areas. Do not expose to a flame.

❑ When transferring substances into other containers, each container must be labeled clearly as to content, procedures for use, and disposal.

Site

❑ There must be sufficient space for girls to move around while working, and space for table work for each girl when appropriate.

❑ Work sites must be well ventilated for activities involving hazardous materials and spray paints (for example, turpentine, spray fixatives, varnishes) or dusts from ceramics.

❑ Flammable material must be used only in work spaces that are removed from ignition sources such as open flames, heaters, and candles.

❑ Provision must be made for proper and safe disposal of all waste materials.

❑ There must be clearly marked fire exits, and fire safety equipment must be on hand.

❑ Food and beverages must not be consumed in activity areas.

Emergency Procedures and First Aid

❑ A first-aid kit must be available.

❑ First-aid procedures must be written, understood, practiced, and posted.

❑ Emergency procedures must be clearly posted for the accidental swallowing of a chemical, or getting a chemical in the eyes, skin contact with a chemical, etc.

National Organizations

Center for Safety in the Arts, National Safety Council.

Backpacking

Planning and Supervision

❑ The leader must have taken council-approved training in teaching backpacking.

❑ The leader must be well versed in "no trace" or "minimal-impact" camping techniques.

❑ A series of conditioning hikes must be planned and conducted before the backpacking trip.

❑ The length of the trip must be determined by the following factors: backpackers' ages, level of experience, physical condition, nature of the terrain, weight of the load to be carried, season and weather conditions, water quantity and quality, and activities planned along the way.

❑ The backpacking party must consist of a minimum of four people, including two adults. The size of the group should be planned to minimize its impact on the environment. (Ideally, if injury occurs, one adult cares for the injured girl while the other adult and one other person seek help.)

❑ There must be one adult in the lead and another at the rear of each group of backpackers.

❑ Backpackers must have a comprehensive understanding of the trip and be adequately prepared regarding all skills and safety practices.

❑ A land management or similar agency must be contacted during the trip planning stages to determine available routes and campsites, recommended group size, water quantity and quality, and permits needed.

❑ Instruction must be given on the safety rules for backpacking, such as staying together in a group, recognizing poisonous plants and biting or stinging insects and ticks, respecting wild animals, and behaving effectively in emergencies.

❑ Group members must be trained to be observant of the route, the surroundings, and the fatigue of individuals.

❑ Each girl must carry a supply of water.

❑ There must be adequate rest periods with time to replenish fluids and to eat high-energy food.

❑ Training must be given in map reading, compass use, route navigation, and estimating distance.

❑ Guidelines must be developed for dealing with problems that may arise with other groups of backpackers.

Clothing

❑ Girls must learn the proper care of their feet, such as treatment for blisters. A thin, smooth sock under a thick sock will reduce friction and absorb perspiration better.

❑ Comfortable, well-broken-in, sturdy walking shoes or ankle-high boots must be worn as appropriate to the terrain.

❑ Soft-soled shoes, such as sneakers, should be worn around the campsite to reduce impact.

❑ Protective clothing appropriate for the weather must be worn.

❑ Clothing must allow girls to move freely and be easily carried when not worn.

Equipment

❑ A complete checklist of group and personal equipment must be made.

❑ Girls must be given instruction on choosing backpacks, adjusting them, making simple repairs, and taking them on and off.

❑ Backpacks and all equipment, food, and water being carried must not weigh more than 20 percent of each person's ideal body weight.

❑ Tents must be flame-resistant. Plastic tents must not be used.

❑ Portable cookstoves must be used whenever possible to reduce the use of wood in back-country areas. See activity checkpoints on Portable Cookstoves.

❑ The foods taken must be nutritious, nonperishable, high-energy, and easily digestible.

❑ Foods must be packaged so as to reduce the number of containers and the amount of trash. See activity checkpoints on Cooking, Food Preparation, and Cleaning.

❑ Water purification supplies must be carried. Water from all natural sources must be considered potentially contaminated and purified before drinking. Water filters used must be designed to remove *Giardia lamblia* from water. See activity checkpoints on Cooking, Food Preparation, and Cleaning.

❑ Plastic bags should be carried for the removal of garbage, used toilet paper and sanitary supplies, etc.

Transportation

❑ Transportation arrangements must be made in advance and confirmed before departure.

Site

❑ The route must be known to one of the adult leaders or a report must be obtained in advance to assess potential hazards.

❑ The route chosen must be within the ability of every girl in the group; the pace must accommodate the slowest hiker.

❑ Camping and fire-building permits must be obtained in advance, if applicable, and carried.

❏ The campsite must be chosen and set up well before dark. Hiking off-trail and after dusk is not recommended.

❏ The group must hike away from the edges of waterfalls, rock ledges, and slopes with loose rocks.

❏ A previously established campsite should be used if available. The campsite must be level and at least 200 feet from all water sources and below treeline. Fragile mountain meadows and areas of wet soil must be avoided. Check overhead and avoid camping under dead tree limbs.

❏ Existing fire rings must be used if a fire is necessary.

❏ If a latrine is not available, individual "cat holes" must be used to dispose of human waste. Cat holes must be at least 200 feet away from the trail and known water sources.

❏ Carry out all garbage, tampons, sanitary supplies, and toilet paper.

❏ Dishes must be washed at least 200 feet away from water sources. Use biodegradable soap. Pour the used water onto soil with good drainage. Remove any food scraps and add them to the garbage being packed out.

❏ Personal bathing and washing must be done at least 200 feet away from water sources. Bury toothpaste spit.

❏ All food must be stored well away from tents and out of the reach of animals. Where necessary, hang food and garbage, used toilet paper, sanitary supplies, etc., at least 10

feet high from a rope stretched between two trees. If the site is in bear country, check with local authorities on precautions to take. (See Hiking activity checkpoints.)

Emergency Procedures and First Aid

❏ An adult with current first-aid training must be present.

❏ A first-aid kit must be taken and equipped with additional supplies such as ace bandages, sunburn remedy, etc.

❏ The itinerary and time schedule must be left at home with a contact person. It must include the route to be taken, the names of the backpackers, the names of the leaders, the activities planned, and the alternate route. The contact person must be called upon departure and upon the return home.

❏ Methods of communication with sources of emergency care, such as police, hospitals, and park and fire officials, must be known and arranged in advance.

❏ Security plans and procedures must be established and shared with backpackers, the council, and appropriate authorities.

❏ The procedures to follow in case of emergencies, such as a search-and-rescue plan, must be written down and reviewed with all participants in advance.

❏ An alternate route must be planned in case of an emergency.

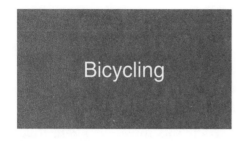

Bicycling

For comfort and safety, girls must have a bicycle of the proper size, and it must be in good condition. Brakes, gears, pedals, chains, seats, and tires should be checked before any day or extended trips.

Planning and Supervision

❏ Instruction must be given by an adult with experience, knowledge, and skill in teaching and/or supervising bicycling.

❏ Girls must be instructed in and practice bicycle-riding skills in traffic, including signaling, scanning ahead and behind—especially before moving left—yielding to oncoming traffic, and making left turns.

❏ The length and terrain for a trip, day or extended, must be appropriate to the girls' skill level, their experience, their physical condition, the time of day, the weather, and the equipment available.

❏ Participants must travel in groups of five to six, allowing at least 150 feet between groups so that vehicles may pass except when on bicycle paths.

❏ For every two groups, there must be an adult at the head and another at the rear.

The following are some general tips and requirements for preparing for a trip and when on the road:

❏ Bike route maps or lists of recommended bike routes that many states publish should be obtained.

❏ The route must be reviewed and map-reading skills must be practiced before departure. Be sure to take the map.

❏ Careful plans must be made for the type of road to be traveled. For example, secondary roads are quiet, and may have trees, curves, and hills that obstruct visibility.

❏ Participants must learn to recognize and avoid common hazards, including vertical drain grates, sand, glass, wet leaves, and litter on shoulders, and other road-surface hazards, to communicate and cooperate with other road users, and to learn to ride in a defensive manner. Motor vehicle traffic presents the greatest danger to cyclists, while stationary hazards such as oil, wet leaves, parked cars, and rocks cause the majority of cycling accidents.

❏ Participants must practice riding their bikes with a load comparable in weight to the load on the trip.

❏ Participants must learn to brake before they have to, especially on curves and downhills. Emergency braking techniques must be taught.

❏ Trips begin and end during the daylight hours.

❏ Participants must cycle single file with traffic; it is acceptable to ride briefly two abreast when passing a slower bicyclist.

❏ Participants must ride with the flow of traffic and obey all applicable traffic regulations, signals, lane markings, and local ordinances pertaining to bicycle operation.

❏ Light gear must be carried in bicycle panniers or packs on the back of the bike.

❏ Bicyclists must make a full stop and look left, right, and left again, especially at the end of a driveway, before entering a street or roadway.

❏ Bicycles must be walked across busy intersections.

❏ Bicycle licenses must be obtained where required (some localities license the bike, not the cyclist).

❏ Girls must use hand signals to indicate turning or stopping.

❏ Bicyclists must not weave in and out of traffic, or between parked cars.

❏ Girls must ride one to a bicycle except when riding tandem. In such cases, each girl must have her own seat and the number of riders should not exceed the intended limits of the bicycle.

❏ A safe distance must be kept between each bicyclist and the vehicle ahead.

❏ Bicycles must have lights and reflectors. Lights should be on to increase visibility when bicycles are not on segregated bicycle paths.

Clothing

❏ Participants must wear comfortable, close-fitting clothing that cannot catch in the gears or the chain; use pant clips or bands if needed.

❏ Participants must wear reflective or very light-colored clothes when cycling at dawn or dusk.

❏ Participants must wear bright-colored or fluorescent clothing during the day.

❏ Participants must wear layers of clothing on extended trips, and carry extra clothes and rain gear.

Equipment

❏ Bicycle helmets must be worn to prevent head injuries. Purchase helmets that meet or exceed the Snell Memorial Foundation or American National Standards Institute (ANSI) Z90.4 standards, as indicated by a sticker inside the helmet.

❏ Helmets must be in good condition and sized properly to fit comfortably but snugly.

❏ A repair kit must be carried. It must contain a pump, tire patch kit, tire irons, screwdriver, adjustable wrench, pliers, and lubricating fluids.

❏ Bicyclists must make sure each bike is in working order, including horn or bell, headlamp, taillight, and reflectors.

Site

❏ All state and local regulations must be observed.

❏ Participants must use designated bicycle trails whenever possible.

❏ Select bicycle trails with even surfaces.

❏ Jurisdictional authorities—for example, highway police—must be notified about the group's trip, when necessary.

❏ The location of emergency services along the route must be known in advance.

❏ A route involving heavily traveled streets and highways must be avoided.

Emergency Procedures and First Aid

❏ An adult with current first-aid training must be present.

❏ A first-aid kit must be available.

❏ Medical services must be available along the selected route.

❏ In the event of an electrical storm, seek low ground and shelter. If a sheltered area is not available, crouch low to the ground in an open area. Stay away from tall, solitary objects such as trees or electrical poles.

❏ A detailed itinerary and an established call-in schedule must be provided for each day.

❏ A list of emergency phone numbers and addresses of bike repair shops must be carried.

❏ Each rider must carry identification on her person at all times.

❏ Each rider must be capable of emergency maneuvers (for example, panic stop, rock dodge, instant turn).

Additional Checkpoints for Bicycle Touring

Safety and comfort on extended bicycle trips demand the use of some essential cycling skills. Long-distance, overnight touring can involve many hours of cycling, sometimes in difficult terrain and with more weight than on day trips. Body conditioning before the tour is important.

❏ Bicycles must be adjusted continuously for comfort. Check the handlebars after adjusting the seat for proper leg extension.

❏ Participants must pad handlebars or wear cycling gloves to soften road vibrations.

❏ Participants must carry two to three water bottles and must drink frequently. Carbonated beverages should be avoided.

❏ Participants should not stop cycling abruptly; cool down gradually by walking around for a few minutes.

❏ Bicyclists must learn to listen to their bodies and not push past the safe level of endurance.

National Organizations

American Youth Hostels, Bicycle Federation of America, Bike-Centennial, National 4H, National Safety Council, U.S. Cycling Federation.

Boating

The guidelines in this section apply to watercraft 26 feet or less in length. For watercraft 26 feet plus in length, see the general tips under "Activity Considerations" (pages 56–59) and "Planning Trips with Girl Scouts" (pages 126–140).

Review the guidelines in this activity checkpoint as well as those for the particular type of craft being used. See checkpoints for:

- Canoeing
- Sailing
- Water skiing
- Windsurfing
- Rafting
- Rowboating
- Tubing
- Sea touring or sea kayaking
- Whitewater kayaking

Whenever possible, it is important for girls to feel safe and confident in the water before participating in activities on the water. To determine each girl's comfort level in the water, conduct a safety exercise such as the following when water temperatures are not prohibitive:

Under the supervision of a certified lifeguard, participants practice putting on a life jacket, entering the water, righting themselves, and coming to the surface. They practice floating and moving with minimal progress.

Planning and Supervision

❑ The boating instructor must have certification or documented experience indicating knowledge and skill in teaching and/or supervising the specific boating activity, e.g., rowboating, flatwater canoeing, whitewater kayaking, sailing, or rafting.

❑ The adult/participant ratio must be appropriate to the boat's size and capacity, the number of boats, the girls' skill and experience, and the water and weather conditions. (See the "Aquatic Supervision Ratios" section, page 56.)

❑ A minimum of two qualified adults must supervise all boating activities.

❑ One adult must be a certified instructor/qualified leader for the type of small craft used.

❑ Instructions on boating safety and emergency procedures must be thoroughly reviewed and practiced while on land, including:

❑ Preventing overloading

❑ Proper distribution of weight

❑ Self-rescue

❑ Preventing heat exhaustion or heatstroke

❑ Preventing hypothermia

❑ Distress signaling

❑ Emergency weather procedures, such as in an electrical storm or high winds

❑ Safe boarding and movement on the craft

❑ Use of emergency equipment

❑ "Rules of the road" for water traffic

❑ General craft handling

❑ Towing procedures

❑ A system that is both audible and visible for recalling craft must be taught in all classes.

❑ On a controlled waterfront, a system must be in place to determine the location of swimmers and boaters, such as a checkboard system.

❑ Craft weight and capacity must not be exceeded; some craft have the maximum capacity clearly displayed. Consider the weather and water conditions, the weight of the passengers, and the equipment.

❑ Marine and weather forecasts must be obtained and monitored for the area in which boating will take place.

Clothing

❑ Laced sneakers or other nonslip footwear designed for water sports must be worn.

Equipment

❑ Boats must be seaworthy, fit for water conditions, and used only for the purposes designed.

❑ Boats must comply with U.S. Coast Guard regulations and/or state and local codes.

❑ **A U.S. Coast Guard-approved personal flotation device (PFD or life jacket) must be worn by each person at all times when boating, regardless of swimming ability.**

❑ Each person must be instructed in the proper use and fit of the PFD that she is wearing.

❑ The use of a PFD must be demonstrated and practiced by each person, preferably including an in-the-water experience with the PFD to test the fit and amount of flotation it provides.

❑ Every PFD must be in serviceable condition and appropriate for the type of waters on which the boat will be used.

❑ Each wearable PFD (Types I, II, III, V, and Hybrid) must be the appropriate size for the person who wears it (within the weight range and chest size marked on the PFD).

❑ At least one graspable and throwable PFD (Type IV buoyant cushion or ring buoy or equivalent) must be immediately available for each group on the water.

❑ PFDs must have whistles attached for signaling purposes when watercraft are used for trips beyond the immediate waterfront area.

❑ All equipment required by federal, state, and local regulations for the particular craft and waters must be aboard, in serviceable condition, and, if appropriate, labeled "U.S. Coast Guard-approved."

❑ No gasoline, liquified petroleum gas, or other types of flammable liquids may be used with heating, cooking, or lighting appliances on board.

❑ A repair kit and tools must be carried as appropriate.

Transportation

❑ The driver must know and use the equipment required by law when trailering a boat.

❑ The driver must learn the principles and master the challenges of driving a tow vehicle and trailer.

Site

When using boating sites that are either council-owned or public, loaned, or donated facilities, the same general principles must be observed in every situation:

❑ Council guidance must be obtained in selecting the boating area.

❑ The swimming area must be separated from the boating area.

❑ Present weather conditions and the long-range forecast must be acceptable.

❑ Water conditions must be suitable (consider currents, tides, presence of dams, water releases, underwater obstructions, etc.).

❑ Visibility must be good.

❑ A lifeboat and rescue equipment must be available where appropriate.

Emergency Procedures and First Aid

❑ An adult with current first-aid training must be present.

❑ A first-aid kit must be available.

❑ The instructors must be qualified to operate all safety and rescue equipment.

❑ A float plan must be filed with local authorities and a back-home contact on shore indicating:

❑ The names of all persons on board

❑ The destination

❑ A description of the craft

❑ The times of departure and return

❑ A list of marine communications, if applicable (VHF radio, Channel 16, is constantly monitored for distress calls and is also used as a contact frequency for all recreational boaters.)

❑ The route to be taken and an alternate route

❑ The agency or person to be notified if return is delayed

❑ Basic emergency procedures for person overboard, rough weather, fire fighting, etc., must be understood and practiced by all.

The basic communication system between the craft and land must be established, such as hand signals, whistles, flags, etc.

Distress signals must be clearly understood.

National Organizations

American Red Cross, U.S. Coast Guard, U.S. Power Squadron.

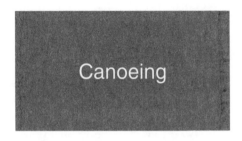

Canoeing

(Also read Boating activity checkpoints.)

Planning and Supervision

Flatwater Canoeing. One adult must be currently certified as a Flatwater, Moving, Paddling, and River Paddling Instructor from the American Canoe Association or in Small Craft Safety from the American Red Cross, or have equivalent certification, or have documented experience indicating knowledge and skill in teaching and/or supervision specific to the canoeing activity conducted.

Whitewater Canoeing. One adult must be currently certified as a Whitewater Instructor from the American Canoe Association or certified in Small Craft Safety with Moving Water module from the American Red Cross, or have equivalent certification, or have documented experience and skills in teaching and/or supervision specific to the canoeing activity.

The adult instructor/trip leader must know the International Scale of River Difficulty and the Universal River Signals from the American Whitewater Affiliation and its Safety Code.

The adult instructor/trip leader must have firsthand knowledge about the hazards and rapids on the river to be run.

The river conditions must be checked on the day the river is to be run. Participants must be instructed how to negotiate the hazards and rapids.

Tripping—Flatwater and Whitewater Canoeing. One adult must be currently certified as a Moving Water Instructor from the American Canoe Association, or certified in Small Craft Safety from the American Red Cross, or have equivalent certification or documented experience indicating knowledge and skill in teaching and/or supervision specific to the trip.

❑ The adult instructor/trip leader must know the International Scale of River Difficulty and the Universal River Signals from the American Whitewater Affiliation and its Safety Code.

❑ A float plan, including an alternate course, if appropriate, must be filed with local authorities and a back-home contact. The authorities and the back-home contact person must be notified upon departure and return. Be prepared to alter the float plan if weather conditions change.

❑ The adult instructor/trip leader must have firsthand knowledge about the hazards and rapids on the river to be run.

❑ The river conditions must be checked on the day the river is to be run. Participants must be instructed how to negotiate the hazards and rapids.

The following apply to all forms of canoeing:

❑ The instructor/qualified leader to participant ratio for canoeing is:

  ❑ 1 to 12 participants for flatwater.

  ❑ 1 to 8 participants for whitewater and tripping.

❑ A minimum of 2 adults must supervise any canoeing activity.

❑ The canoeing skills of the adults must be higher than the difficulty of the intended activity or trip.

❑ Each girl's comfort level in the water must be assessed as described in the Boating activity checkpoints on page 70 before going canoeing.

❑ Canoeing activities conducted on whitewater or semiprotected waters must meet the Safety Code of the American Whitewater Affiliation.

Clothing

❑ For protection against hypothermia, a wetsuit may be worn when the water temperature is below 50°F. When the combined air and water temperature is less than 100°F, or when the combination of cool air, wind chill, and evaporative cooling may lead to hypothermia, a wetsuit may be worn. Dressing in layers—using wool, nylon, or polypropylene pile under a paddling jacket and pants made of a coated material to repel water—will help to protect the body from getting chilled.

❑ Sneakers or other adequate foot protection must be worn while paddling.

Equipment

❑ Each person must wear a PFD.

❑ Canoes 15 feet or less in length—no more than 2 persons.

❑ All persons must wear a safety helmet in Class III waters or above.

❑ The safety helmet must be a properly fitted, flexible, strong, plastic shell with a chin strap and openings for drainage.

❑ Craft weight and capacity must not be exceeded. Consider the weather and water conditions, the weight of the passengers, and the equipment.

❑ All canoes must have a painter (also called end line or grab line) secured to each end of the canoe. A painter must be a strong line that floats, and must be at least half the length of the canoe.

❑ Paddles must be in good repair and sized to each canoeist. On longer trips or those involving whitewater, one extra paddle per canoe must be carried.

❑ For trips of 48 hours or less on flatwater, two or three extra paddles must be carried by each group. For trips of over 48 hours, one extra paddle per canoe must be carried by each group.

❑ For river rescue, each instructor/leader must attach a locking blade knife, two carabiners, and two prusik loops to her/his PFD or secure them to the canoe in an easily accessible place. (The prusik loop is a type of mountaineering knot with loops used with a carabiner for quick tie-offs and z-drag rescues, which use a pulley system to recover a canoe pinned against a rock or other obstacle.)

❑ Additional gear (clothing, sleeping, cooking) must be stored in waterproof containers or packages and secured in the canoe. **Do not overload the canoe.**

Transportation

❑ Canoes must be transported on car-top racks or canoe trailers. Canoes must be secured with two lines across the top and a line bow and stern.

Site

❑ Council guidance must be obtained in selecting canoeing sites.

❑ No canoeing shall be done on water that has not been run and rated.

❑ No canoeing shall be taken on whitewater more difficult than Class IV as defined by the American Version of the International Scale of River Difficulty. However, rivers may be run where short stretches of Class IV waters are negotiated if the girls have the proper skills, are well supervised, and if the option always exists to carry around the rapids.

Emergency Procedures and First Aid

❑ One adult with current first-aid training must be present.

❑ A first-aid kit must be kept within reach of the first-aider. The first-aid kit must be kept in a waterproof container and secured in the canoe.

❑ First-aid procedures must be reviewed, including those for immersion hypothermia, near-drowning, sprains, and fractures.

❑ Arrangements must be made in advance for medical emergencies and evacuation procedures.

❏ During storms, if shore cannot be reached, secure all loose gear, keep a sharp lookout for other boats and obstructions, head into the wind at a 45° angle and stay low.

❏ An emergency survival packet that includes items such as waterproof matches, emergency food supplies, a flashlight and extra batteries, and a lightweight emergency blanket used to retain body heat must be taken on all trips.

National Organizations

American Canoe Association, American Red Cross, American Whitewater Affiliation, National Organization for River Sports, United States Canoe Association.

Challenge Courses

Challenge courses are not recommended for Daisy Girl Scouts. Brownie Girl Scouts can take part in components of the challenge course that are not off the ground.

A challenge (or teams) course is a set of structures that provide a setting for physical challenges designed to increase participant self-confidence and physical coordination, to increase group cooperation, and to have fun. Activities done on structures **less** than six feet off the ground must follow these checkpoints. For activities done more than six feet off the ground, see the checkpoints for Ropes Courses and Rappelling in *Safety and Risk Management in Girl Scouting*.

Planning and Supervision

❏ An instructor who has successfully completed a training workshop in the proper use of the course and group process techniques must directly supervise the group.

❏ No more than 10 participants should be assigned to each instructor. In activities involving Brownie Girl Scouts, no more than five participants should be assigned to each instructor. At least two instructors must be present.

❏ Before each use, the instructor must inspect all equipment and landing areas.

❏ Instructors must be skilled in selecting appropriate sites for activities, teaching spotting techniques, and modifying tasks to provide an appropriate experience for the group.

❏ The instructor must describe the objectives, safety procedures, and potential health and safety risks to the group before beginning an activity. A debriefing must follow the activity.

❏ Spotting techniques must be taught, demonstrated, and practiced by participants. All activities must be appropriately spotted. In activities where Brownie Girl Scouts take part, the spotters must be adults.

❏ Girls must not be pushed beyond their capabilities nor forced to participate.

❑ Participants must not be stacked more than three levels high vertically on each other at any one time. No one should stand in the middle of someone else's back.

❑ For activities where partners are needed, instructors must match participants according to size and skill level, if necessary.

❑ All participants must participate in muscle warm-up and stretching activities before beginning strenuous physical activities.

Clothing

❑ All instructors and participants must wear sturdy shoes and long pants.

❑ Objects in pockets and around necks and fingers must be removed and eyeglasses removed or secured. Large or sharp belts must be removed. Long hair must be pulled back from the face and fastened to prevent loose ends from tangling.

Equipment

❑ Safety helmets designed for rock climbing must be worn on rock sites. Climbing helmets must have the UIAA-approved label (Union of International Alpine Associations).

Site

❑ Before using a non-Girl Scout facility, council approval must be obtained.

❑ The facility must be appropriate to the skill and ability level of the girls.

❑ If structures are provided, the site must be planned and constructed by experienced individuals.

❑ The site must be free of obvious hazards.

❑ The site must not be used in hazardous weather conditions.

❑ The site must be planned with minimal disturbance to the natural environment.

❑ Safety rules must be written, practiced, and posted in the area.

❑ Plans and procedures must be established to avoid unauthorized use of the site, structures, and equipment. The site must be posted to warn against unauthorized use.

Emergency Procedures and First Aid

❑ An adult with current first-aid training must be present.

❑ A first-aid kit must be available along with equipment appropriate to the activity.

❑ A written safety plan must be established and practiced.

❑ Emergency transportation must be available.

National Organization

Association for Experiential Education.

Community Activities and Events

These include service projects, parades, large group gatherings, and so forth.

Planning and Supervision

❑ The Girl Scout council must be contacted for approval and guidance before participating in any community activities or events.

❑ The appropriateness of the activity or event must be considered, including:

- ❑ The needs, interests, and readiness of the girls
- ❑ The sponsor
- ❑ The needs of the community to be served
- ❑ Scheduling concerns
- ❑ Possible environmental and health risks
- ❑ GSUSA and council guidelines on fund raising, endorsements, collaborating with other organizations, and maintaining nonprofit status

❑ Local regulations and permit procedures must be observed relating to public gatherings, facility use, food handling, certificates of insurance, sales or excise tax, etc.

❑ Adult supervision must be sufficient in terms of age of participants, event size, security arrangements, and time of day (see Program Standard 13).

❑ The location of girls must be known at all times by the leaders.

❑ Instruction must be given on safe pedestrian practices, when applicable.

❑ Guidelines for personal protection must be observed. Local authorities must be contacted for safety and security suggestions and assistance applicable to the project, event, or parade.

❑ GSUSA and council guidelines on publicity, photo releases, etc., must be observed.

❑ Girls must be released to no one other than a legal parent or guardian, unless other arrangements were made in writing prior to the event.

❑ Arrangements for picking up the girls after the event must be made in advance and clearly described for parents and girls.

❑ Leaders and girls must discuss a "lost plan" and set a place to meet in case of separation from the adult in charge or from the group.

Clothing

❑ Girls must wear the Girl Scout pin and/or some means of group identification.

❑ Name tags or other personal identification must not be worn in public places for safety reasons.

❑ Comfortable shoes and socks must be worn for long walks and parades.

Transportation

❑ All transporation for events must be managed in a safe manner, following Program Standards 25 and 26 for Private Transportation and Public Transportation.

The following points regarding floats must be adhered to:

❑ Floats drawn by trucks and automobiles must be covered by automobile insurance in the name of owners of the vehicles.

❑ Float construction must be safe, using no toxic or highly flammable materials, and be secured to the body of the float and the vehicle.

❑ Floats must be equipped with portable ABC fire extinguishers.

❑ Riders on floats must be provided with secure seating, a secure handhold, or a safety harness if standing.

❑ Floats must not be overcrowded.

❑ Participants must not walk close to moving floats.

❑ An adult must accompany girls on any moving float.

❑ The driver of the float must eliminate any blind spot hazards.

❑ Any coupling of a trailer to a vehicle must be appropriate to the load and have a safety chain.

❑ Nothing may be distributed to onlookers from a moving vehicle or float.

Site

❑ The location for any community event, large group gathering, or parade must be inspected in advance, with consideration for the following, as they apply:

❑ Accessibility to the group and to the public

❑ Suitability to event size, age groups, and kinds of activities

❑ Parking availability

❑ Availability of restrooms

❑ Security arrangements

❑ Lighting for evening and indoor events

❑ Vulnerability to inclement weather

❑ Proximity to medical facilities

❑ Availability of police protection

❑ Potential for environmental or health risks

❑ Fire safety

❑ The occupancy limits must not be exceeded for indoor gatherings and events.

❑ Emergency exits must be sufficient, well marked, and operational.

❑ Any food preparation area used for large groups of people must meet state and local standards.

❑ Sufficient potable water and restrooms must be made available to participants.

❑ Provisions must be made for garbage removal and site cleanup.

❑ All other basic safety and security guidelines must be followed (see pages 11–28).

Emergency Procedures and First Aid

❑ There must be a designated first-aid station with an adult currently trained in first-aid present.

❑ A first-aid kit must be available.

❑ An emergency vehicle must be available at large group gatherings.

❑ Location of the nearest telephone must be known at all times.

❑ The leader must carry emergency contact telephone numbers.

❑ An evacuation plan must be part of written and oral communication with participants for any large indoor or outdoor gathering.

National Organization

National Safety Council.

Cookie/Council-Sponsored Product Sales

Daisy Girl Scouts may not participate in cookie or other product sales.

Planning and Supervision

❑ Council guidelines must be observed.

❑ Local ordinances related to involvement of children in money-earning projects must be observed.

❑ Girls must be involved in planning and setting goals for the product sale.

❑ Each girl's participation must be voluntary.

❑ Written permission must be obtained from a girl's parent or guardian before the girl participates in a council product sale.

❑ Adult supervision and guidance are essential during each step of the sale. A parent or other adult must know each girl's whereabouts when she is engaged in product sales.

Clothing

❑ Girls must be identifiable as Girl Scouts by wearing a membership pin or uniform or carrying a membership card.

Order Taking and Selling

❑ Girls must be familiar with the areas and neighborhoods in which they will sell.

❑ Adults must monitor, supervise, and guide all age levels. Adults must accompany Brownie and Junior Girl Scouts.

❏ Girls may participate in door-to-door sales only when accompanied by an adult.

❏ The buddy system must be used.

❏ When Girl Scouts operate a booth in a store, mall, or other public place, an adult must be present at all times.

❏ Girls must learn and practice personal protection skills as outlined in their handbooks. For example:

  ❏ Do not enter the home of a stranger.

  ❏ Use safe pedestrian practices, especially when crossing at busy intersections.

  ❏ Do not carry large amounts of money.

  ❏ Provisions for safeguarding the money must be made in advance. Adult support assures that girls are not carrying large sums of money.

❏ The troop leader's or designated telephone number must be given for reorders or complaints; a girl must not give her telephone number.

❏ When planning sales outlets, contact local authorities for permission as well as for additional safety and security suggestions and assistance.

Emergency Procedures and First Aid

❏ An itinerary must be left with a contact person.

❏ Security plans and procedures must be established and known.

Cooking, Food Preparation, and Cleaning

This activity checkpoint applies to outdoor cooking.

Planning and Supervision

❏ Instruction must be given in the safe use of kitchen tools and equipment, such as knives, grinders, and mixers.

❏ Health considerations must be reviewed, including the importance of keeping utensils and hands clean, cooking meats thoroughly, refrigerating perishables, etc.

❏ Meals must be nutritionally sound, reflect girl planning, take into account food allergies, and consider the religious and dietary beliefs of group members.

❏ Any person with a skin infection, cold, or communicable disease must not be involved in food preparation.

❏ Whenever possible, buy food and supplies that avoid excess packaging, and buy in bulk.

❏ Recycle whenever possible.

❏ Cooking facilities must be adequate to avoid overcrowding.

❑ Discipline must be maintained around the campfire and stove and in areas where knives or other tools are being used.

Equipment

❑ The manufacturer's instructions for cookstoves must be followed.

❑ All equipment, containers, and cooking utensils used to prepare food must be kept clean.

❑ When dishes are washed by hand, use the following procedures:

   ❑ Remove food particles from utensils and dishes.

   ❑ Wash in warm, soapy water.

   ❑ Rinse in hot, clear water.

❑ Sanitize by one of the following methods:

   ❑ Rinse in clear, boiling water or

   ❑ Immerse for at least one minute in a sanitizing solution approved by the local health department.

❑ Air-dry and store in a clean, covered area.

❑ Dishwashing and rinse water must be disposed of according to the regulations of the campsite. Waste water must be disposed of at least 200 feet beyond any water source or trail.

❑ Potholders or pot grippers must be used to prevent burns.

❑ Unbreakable containers must be used outdoors.

❑ Chipped or cracked items, such as glass, enamel, or plastic dishes, must not be used.

❑ Each person must have an individual drinking cup.

❑ Food must be stored in a manner that prevents spoilage and contamination.

❑ Perishables such as creamed dishes, pudding, dairy products, poultry, meats, and salads must be stored at or below 45°F in a refrigerator or insulated cooler with ice enclosed. If this temperature cannot be maintained for food storage, use powdered, dehydrated, freeze-dried, or canned goods.

❑ Foods requiring refrigeration must not be used on extended camping trips.

❑ Safe water must be used to reconstitute powdered, dehydrated, or freeze-dried food. Once reconstituted, any perishable items must be eaten within one hour or refrigerated.

❑ Food must be stored well away from tents and sleeping quarters, and out of the reach of animals. Where necessary, hang food at least 10 feet high from a rope stretched between two trees. If the site is in bear territory, check with local authorities on precautions to take.

Site

❑ The current weather conditions must be suitable for fire building or the use of an outdoor cookstove.

❑ All food preparation surfaces and dining areas must be kept clean.

❑ When there is a campsite garbage pickup service, garbage must be stored in a tight, insect- and animal-proof container with plastic inner lining, and covered securely.

❑ When there is no garbage pickup service, separate all refuse according to instructions at the site.

❑ Do not bury food.

❑ All grease must be carried out.

❑ Food containers and cans must be rinsed before discarding.

❑ All garbage must be removed from the campsite in plastic bags and discarded as appropriate, or recycled whenever possible.

❑ There must be a safe drinking water supply for cooking, drinking, and personal use. Safe drinking water is defined as water from a tap that has been tested and approved by the local health department. All other sources are considered potentially contaminated.

Emergency Procedures and First Aid

❑ A first-aid kit must be available.

❑ First-aid procedures for burns and cuts must be reviewed.

See also the activity checkpoints for Cooking Fires and for Portable Cookstoves.

Cooking Fires

Portable cookstoves are recommended in day, troop, core, or resident camp settings to conserve wood and shorten cooking time. In many situations, cookstoves are now preferred in primitive camping areas where wood is in short supply. They are required in some areas where groups may be backpacking, horsepacking, or canoe tripping. (See activity checkpoints for Portable Cookstoves, pages 94–95.)

Planning and Supervision

❑ The instructor must have taken council training in teaching and/or supervising cooking fires.

❑ Instruction must be provided for fire-building and fire safety skills.

❏ Local and state regulations must be observed. Check with the local fire district, land management agency, or conservation office to see whether a permit is required.

❏ The type of fire planned must be appropriate for the meal and the experience of the girl.

❏ Discipline around the fire site must be maintained.

❏ The following rules must be observed for open wood or charcoal fires:

    ❏ One instructor must be present when the fire is lit.

    ❏ Keep the fire small.

    ❏ Do not crowd around the fire.

    ❏ Store wood and charcoal away from the fire area.

    ❏ Watch for flying sparks and put them out immediately.

    ❏ A bucket of water, soil, or sand must be on hand to extinguish the fire.

    ❏ The fire must be completely out before leaving the site. To be sure, sprinkle the fire with water or smother it with earth or sand. Then stir, and sprinkle or smother again. Finally, check by holding hands over coals, ashes, or partially burned wood or charcoal for one minute. It should be cool to the touch.

❏ Plan to use use alternative sources of fuel whenever possible, such as propane, butane, gasoline, charcoal, and buddy burners.

Clothing

❏ Dangling or loose clothing or accessories must not be worn near a fire. Roll up long sleeves, tie back long hair, and do not wear plastic garments, such as ponchos, around an open flame.

Equipment

❏ Matches must be stored in a waterproof container.

❏ Long-handled cooking utensils and pot holders or pot grippers must be used to protect hands when cooking.

❏ Cooking pots must not be overfilled.

❏ Fire-fighting equipment must be available, including water, loose soil or sand, and a shovel and rake.

❏ Pressurized cans, plastic basins, bottles, and cooking utensils must not be used near a fire.

❏ A candle or similar fire starter must be used as a means to conserve matches, especially in inclement weather.

❏ Charcoal fires must never be started with gasoline.

❏ Dispose of burned coals as per site regulations.

Site

❏ A fire permit, where applicable, should be secured for a fire. Fires are not permitted where there is excessive dryness or wind. Check the fire index with local land management agencies or the fire district or consult the radio.

❏ Fires must be built in designated areas. Avoid establishing new fire sites, if possible.

❏ An established fire site must be away from overhanging branches, steep slopes, rotted stumps or logs, dry grass and leaves, and cleared of any burnable material, such as litter, duff, or pine needles.

❏ An established fire site must have a five-foot radius around a small fire; in dry and windy areas, a seven-foot radius around the fire must be observed.

❏ Sensitivity toward the environment must be shown:

  ❏ Clean the fire site. Preserve the natural beauty of the site and surrounding area before leaving.

  ❏ Follow local air pollution regulations.

  ❏ Make economical use of wood. Where wood gathering is permitted, only dead, fallen wood may be used for small cooking fires.

  ❏ A plan for disposal of cold ashes and partially burned wood must be made. Ashes and partially burned wood may be scattered throughout the woods away from the campsite.

❏ Paper trash may be burned only if it can be entirely consumed by fire and only if regulations permit.

Emergency Procedures and First Aid

❏ An adult currently trained in first aid must be present.

❏ A first-aid kit must be available.

❏ Fire safety rules, emergency procedures, and first aid for burns must be reviewed with the group and understood.

❏ Procedures must be established and known in advance for notifying the fire department or land management agency officials in case of a fire.

❏ Fire drills must be practiced periodically.

❏ Plans for evacuation must be discussed in advance and reviewed at the campsite.

See activity checkpoints for Cooking, Food Preparation, and Cleaning and for Portable Cookstoves.

Hayrides

Planning and Supervision

❏ The hayride must be supervised by adults in the appropriate ratio. (See Program Standard 25.)

Transportation

❏ Girls must not ride in the hauling vehicle.

❏ The driver of the hauling vehicle must be licensed to drive a vehicle in the jurisdiction and be at least 21 years of age.

❏ The hauled vehicle must meet all state and local safety requirements and display proper identification showing that these conditions have been met.

❏ The hauled vehicle must have protective sides and rear fencing or gates, as well as rear lights that are in working order.

❏ The hay or straw must be properly stacked to prevent slipping.

❏ Sufficient seating space must be allowed for each person.

❏ Girls and adults must remain seated during the ride.

Site

❏ The hayride must take place on private property at a speed not to exceed 10 miles per hour. Public roads and highways must not be used because slow-moving vehicles can cause serious accidents on roads traveled by automobiles.

National Organization

National Safety Council.

Hiking

This checkpoint does not apply to short walks.

Planning and Supervision

❏ Hikes must be restricted to a reasonable length as determined by age, level of experience, nature of the terrain, physical condition of the hikers, weather conditions, and time of day. Hiking after dusk is not recommended.

❏ Whenever possible, stay on hiking trails. Girls must stay on the pathway to avoid trampling trailside plants and causing erosion.

❏ The buddy system must be used.

❏ The hiking party must consist of a minimum of four people, including two adults. The size of the group should be planned to minimize its impact on the environment. (If injury occurs, one person cares for the patient while the other two seek help.)

❏ There must be one adult in the lead and another adult at the rear of each group of hikers.

❏ Instructions must be given on the safety rules for hiking.

❏ Girls must be instructed in how to adjust packs.

❏ Girls must learn the proper care of their feet, such as treatment for blisters. A thin, smooth sock under a thick sock will reduce friction and absorb perspiration.

❏ Each participant should carry water to drink.

❏ There must be adequate rest periods with time to replenish fluids and to eat high-energy food.

❏ Guidelines must be developed for dealing with problems that may arise with other groups of hikers.

Clothing

❏ Comfortable, well-broken-in, sturdy walking shoes or ankle-high boots must be worn that are appropriate to the terrain.

❏ Protective clothing appropriate for the weather must be worn.

❏ Clothing must allow girls to move freely and be easily carried when not worn.

Transportation

❏ Transportation arrangements must be made in advance and confirmed before departure.

Site

❏ The route must be known to one of the adult leaders or a report must be obtained in advance to assess potential hazards such as poisonous plants, dangerous animals, unsafe drinking water, cliffs, drop-offs, etc. Unsafe routes must not be taken.

❏ The route chosen must be within the ability of every girl in the group; the pace must accommodate the slowest hiker.

❏ Terrain, mileage, and hiking time must be known to the hikers in advance.

❏ The weather report must be known before leaving and monitored during the hike.

❏ Respect for the environment must be demonstrated. Avoid eating wild foods, uprooting or walking on plants, interfering with or feeding wild animals, or littering.

❏ If a latrine is not available, individual "cat holes" must be used to dispose of human waste. Cat holes must be at least 200 feet away from the trail or water source. Carry out all tampons, sanitary supplies, and toilet paper.

Emergency Procedures and First Aid

❏ An adult with current first-aid training must be present.

❏ A first aid-kit must be taken on the hike and equipped with additional supplies, such as ace bandages, sunburn remedy, etc.

❏ The first-aider must be prepared to handle cases of hypothermia, blisters, sprains, fractures, insect stings and tick bites, snake bites, sunburn, and heat- and cold-related illnesses.

❑ The itinerary and time schedule must be left at home with a contact person, and must include the route to be taken, the names of the hikers, the names of the leaders, the activities planned, and the alternate route. The contact person must be called upon departure and upon the return home.

❑ Methods of communication with sources of emergency care, such as police, hospitals, park officials, and fire officials, must be known and arranged in advance.

❑ A search-and-rescue plan for lost hikers must be written down and understood by everyone in advance.

❑ Security plans and procedures must be established and shared with hikers, the council, appropriate authorities, etc.

❑ The procedures to follow in case of emergencies must be written down and reviewed in advance.

National Organizations

Appalachian Mountain Club, Appalachian Trail Conference.

Horseback Riding

To participate in riding, girls must possess physical coordination and balance. They must be old enough to understand and practice safety procedures and to use good judgment in reacting to situations. Girls must be mature enough to take responsibility for themselves and their horses.

Horseback riding is not recommended for Daisy Girl Scouts.

Planning and Supervision

❑ All riding instructors must be adults currently certified by an accredited horsemanship instructor training organization or have documented proof of a minimum of three years' experience successfully instructing in a general horseback riding program.

❑ All assistant riding instructors must be 16 or older and be currently certified by an accredited horsemanship instructor training organization or have documented proof of one year's experience successfully instructing in a general horseback riding program.

❑ Riders must be supervised by instructors or assistant instructors at all times when in the proximity of horses, whether mounted or not.

❑ Each rider must be tested and classified according to her riding ability.

❑ The horse and riding area must be assigned according to the rider's ability.

❑ Beginning riders must attend an introductory safety lesson, including information on horse psychology and behavior, and approaching, handling, and leading a horse.

☐ A beginning rider must ride only in a ring or corral; a rider must feel confident and demonstrate basic skills in controlling the horse and maintaining proper distance before trail riding.

☐ A safety check of each rider's clothing, the horse's tack, and the riding area must be made before each riding session by an instructor.

☐ Only one rider is allowed on a horse at any time.

☐ Eating or drinking is not permitted while riding.

Additional Checkpoints for Ring or Corral Riding

☐ A minimum of one instructor and one assistant instructor must supervise any group of 10 or fewer riders, with one additional instructor or assistant instructor for every five additional riders.

☐ A preride demonstration must be given to all first-time riders, including mounting, dismounting, starting, stopping, steering, and balanced body position.

☐ Each horse and rider must be under the observation of one of the instructors at all times.

Additional Checkpoints for Trail Riding

☐ No more than 10 girls to a group, excluding an instructor and assistant instructor. For beginning riders or younger girls, adult supervision may need to be increased.

☐ Prior to the trail ride, a brief warm-up must take place in a ring or corral to ensure that riders are well suited to their horses, and can control all of the gaits and functions required during the trail ride.

☐ The group must ride single file, one full horse length apart, with the assistant instructor at the head, the least experienced riders in the front, and the instructor at the rear.

☐ Distances between horses must be increased when the horses' speed increases.

☐ Riders must have control of their horses and maintain the spacing between horses.

☐ The length of the trail ride and the gait of the horses must be geared to the ability of the least experienced rider.

☐ Supervision must be increased for inexperienced riders or difficult trails.

☐ Riding trails must have good footing and be free from dangerous obstructions, such as low-hanging branches.

☐ Trails must be marked, mapped, regularly inspected, and maintained.

☐ Gates must be left as found, open or shut.

☐ Public roads and highways must be avoided whenever possible. (If a group must cross a road, the instructors must first halt the group in a line well before the road, check for traffic, and then signal the group to cross. At the signal, all horses are turned to face the highway and all cross at the same time.)

☐ Horses must be walked up and down hills and should be walked for the final 10 minutes of any riding period.

☐ Equipment for a trail ride must include helmets, halters, lead ropes, and rain gear.

☐ Gear must be tied to the saddle or packed in saddlebags. Backpacks, day packs, fanny packs, etc., are not to be worn by any riders.

Other Situations

☐ In case of other horseback riding situations, such as open range riding, horse shows, led pony rides, etc., a written safety management plan specific to the activity must be prepared.

☐ Some programs, such as riding for girls with disabilities, vaulting, pack trips, driving, and games, may require special equipment, as well as horses and instructors with specialized training.

Clothing

☐ Long pants and appropriate protective clothing must be worn.

☐ Clothing must be snug to prevent becoming tangled with the saddle.

☐ Jewelry, especially loop earrings, heavy pendants, and bracelets, must not be worn.

☐ Boots or shoes with at least a half-inch heel must be worn to prevent

feet from sliding through the stirrups.

☐ If tappaderos, a covering across the front of the stirrup that holds the foot in, are used, then an athletic shoe with nonskid sole and ties may be worn.

☐ Riders may not ride in hiking boots with lug soles, tennis shoes, sandals, or barefoot.

☐ Riders may wear well-fitting gloves to protect hands from blisters, rope burns, and cuts.

Equipment

☐ Protective headgear with a properly fitting safety harness that meets the American Society for Testing and Materials (ASTM) F-1163-88 requirements, displaying the Safety Equipment Institute (SEI) seal, must be worn by girls and adults, including all instructors, wranglers, stable hands, etc., when around horses, whether mounted or not.

☐ All equipment must be in good condition, checked regularly for wear, and repaired as necessary.

☐ Records of repair requests and completion of repairs must be maintained and kept.

☐ All equipment must be properly adjusted for each rider and horse.

☐ The saddle size must be appropriate for each rider.

☐ All girth straps must be fitted properly and checked by the instructor prior to mounting.

☐ Stirrup lengths must be adjusted for each rider.

Site

❑ Council approval must be obtained when selecting a non-Girl Scout riding facility.

❑ The stable operator must provide evidence of liability insurance and references from other youth group users of the stable.

❑ The stable area must be inspected prior to use by council staff.

The following applies to both Girl Scout council and non-Girl Scout riding facilities:

❑ The riding area must be away from outside distractions and free of debris.

❑ The barn and riding areas must not have exposed barbed wire fencing.

❑ The instructional rings, corrals, paddocks, and stables must have clearly posted rules and regulations.

❑ The horses must be properly cared for and the stables, corrals, barns, etc., must be kept clean and uncluttered.

❑ Tack (saddles, bridles, etc.) must be clean and in good condition.

❑ Weather conditions must be suitable for riding. The ground must be firm and free of ice.

❑ Riding should be done during daylight hours only. Any riding at night must be in an enclosed, well-lighted area.

❑ Permission and any necessary permits must be obtained before riding on public or private lands.

Emergency Prodedures and First Aid

❑ An adult with current first-aid training must be present in the ring or on the trail.

❑ A first-aid kit must be available in the ring or on the trail.

❑ An emergency vehicle must be readily available.

❑ Plans for emergency communication with the police, hospitals, and park or fire officials must be arranged in advance and known by each instructor.

❑ Plans for response in case of an emergency, such as a fire, severe weather, injured rider, injured or loose horse, etc., must be known by all participants and instructors.

❑ For extended trips, the itinerary must be left with a contact person. The person must be called upon departure and return.

❑ At Girl Scout facilities, a method of communication between the riding area and the site director or health-care personnel must be available.

❑ In stable and ring areas telephone numbers for the fire department, local hospital or emergency ambulance service, and veterinarian must be conspicuously posted, and the location of the fire alarm must be known to all girls and adults.

National Organizations

CHA: The Association for Horsemanship Safety and Education, Horsemanship Safety Association, U.S. Pony Clubs.

Ice Skating

Planning and Supervision

Ice Skating Rink:

❑ Girls should receive basic instruction in ice skating skills and in safety and conduct rules from an experienced ice skating instructor.

❑ Leaders must supervise from outside the main skating floor. (Check with the rink manager in advance to learn how many adults, in addition to the rink staff, are needed to supervise the group.)

❑ Practice sessions must be scheduled for beginners.

❑ The rink manager must be called in advance to arrange for large groups or for practice sessions.

❑ The rink must be adequately staffed to monitor the size and behavior of the crowd.

❑ Girls must learn to perform basic skating skills before attempting more advanced skills.

❑ Girls must learn how to fall and get up correctly as a beginning skill.

❑ Warm-up exercises must be done before any strenuous ice skating; cool-down exercises must end the sessions.

❑ Ice skaters must be instructed on safety rules by the leader or rink manager or both. The rules of the rink must be observed. For example:

 ❑ Everyone must skate in the same direction.

 ❑ Girls should not stop in the main skating area.

 ❑ Skaters must yield the right-of-way to those already in the rink.

 ❑ Skaters must not cut across the paths of other skaters.

 ❑ Skaters must not push, shove, or race on the ice.

 ❑ A falling skater must not grab hold of another skater.

 ❑ A fallen skater must rise quickly, unless injured.

 ❑ Loose or sharp articles, such as handbags, combs, keys, etc., must not be carried in pockets, hands, hair, or anyplace where they might fall to the ice or injure a falling ice skater.

Outdoor Ice Skating:

❑ Girls must ice skate on a pond or lake when supervised, but never on a stream.

❑ Adults supervising the skating area must consult with the park personnel, local police, etc., to determine whether the ice thickness is safe for skating.

❑ Girls must never ice-skate alone; use the buddy system.

❑ Girls may skate at night if the area is well lit.

Clothing

❑ Clothing must allow freedom of movement. Several warm layers are recommended, including hats and gloves or mittens. Bring a change of socks.

Equipment

❑ Girls must receive instruction in selecting the proper skate size.

❑ Ice skates must be properly fitted, securely laced, and properly tied.

❑ Guards must be put on ice skates when girls are not on the ice.

Site

❑ Council guidance must be obtained in selecting the ice skating site. Rinks are the safest place to skate.

Ice Skating Rink:

❑ A rink must have a smooth skating surface free from papers, candy wrappers, and other debris.

❑ The rink safety rules must be posted or announced, or both, and practiced.

Outdoor Ice Skating:

❑ Skating surfaces must be checked in advance for thickness, patches of grass, rocks, cracks, etc.

❑ A list of emergency telephone numbers, including a nearby physician, ambulance, hospital, police, and fire or rescue unit, must be posted or carried by the adult in charge.

❑ Safety rules must be written, reviewed, practiced, and posted.

❑ Appropriate rescue and first-aid equipment must be on hand (e.g., ring buoy, rope, throw bag, pole, ladder, boat).

Emergency Procedures and First Aid

Ice Skating Rink:

❑ The leader must check in advance to see if an adult currently trained in first aid will be available. If not, an adult with current first-aid training must be present.

❑ A first-aid kit must be available.

Outdoor Ice Skating:

❑ An adult with current first-aid training must be present.

❑ A first-aid kit must be available.

❑ The first-aider must be prepared to handle cases of near-drowning and immersion hypothermia.

❑ Basic ice rescue techniques must be understood and practiced.

National Organizations

Ice Skating Institute of America, Professional Skaters Guild of America.

Portable Cookstoves

Portable cookstoves are available in a wide range of sizes and differ in fuel use and safety factors.

Portable cookstoves are encouraged in day, troop, core, or resident camp settings to conserve wood and shorten cooking time. In many situations, cookstoves are now preferred in primitive camping areas where wood is in short supply. They are required in some areas where groups may be backpacking, horsepacking, or canoe tripping.

Fuels for stoves include butane, propane, kerosene, ethyl alcohol, sterno, and gasoline. The manufacturer's instructions for ignition and burning must be followed carefully. Girls must be closely supervised when using any stove, especially when using gasoline, which is highly volatile when used improperly.

Planning and Supervision

☐ Local regulations must be observed. Check with the fire department or land management agency when planning a trip to find out if fires or cookstoves are permitted.

☐ Take an adequate amount of fuel.

☐ The manufacturer's instructions must be carefully followed. Practice with instructions before using with girls.

☐ Portable cookstoves must **never** be used inside a tent or indoors.

☐ All stove parts must be kept clean; see that lines and burners are not clogged.

☐ The cookstove must **never** be refueled or canisters changed near an open flame.

☐ Care must be taken not to spill fuel. If fuel does spill, relocate the stove before lighting.

☐ Avoid overcrowding around the stove.

☐ Girls must not reach over the stove. Determine the best way to stir the contents of the pot without tipping over the pot or stove, or remove the pot from the stove to stir the contents.

Clothing

☐ Long hair should be tied back.

☐ Loose clothing should not be worn around an open flame.

Equipment

☐ Matches must be stored in a waterproof container and kept separate from the stove and fuel supply.

☐ An insulated glove, potholder, or pot gripper must be used to protect hands while cooking.

☐ All portable cookstoves must be placed in safe, level, and stable positions, shielded from the wind and away from foot traffic.

☐ Rocks or other items must not be piled around the cookstove for stability.

☐ The fuel tank must not be overheated.

❏ The pots used must be of appropriate size so that the stove is not top-heavy.

❏ The extra fuel supply must be stored away from the cooking flame.

❏ Pressurized cans must not be disposed of in a fire, placed in direct sunlight, or kept in enclosed areas where the temperature is high. See the manufacturer's instructions on the label. All fuel canisters must be disposed of in the recommended manner.

❏ Fires should be extinguished before retiring for sleep.

❏ Fire-fighting equipment must be on hand, such as a trowel, loose earth, and baking soda, to douse a fire in case of an accident.

Site

❏ The site chosen for the cookstove must be cleared of flammable materials in case the stove tips over or the fuel spills.

❏ The chosen site must be sheltered from the wind.

❏ All fuel canisters and evidence of cooking must be removed from the site. The site must be returned to its original condition.

Emergency Procedures and First Aid

❏ An adult with current first-aid training must be present.

❏ A first-aid kit must be available.

❏ Fire safety rules, emergency procedures, and first aid for burns must be reviewed with the group and understood.

❏ Procedures must be established and known in advance for notifying the fire department or land management agency officials in case of a fire.

❏ Fire drills must be practiced periodically.

❏ Plans for evacuation must be discussed in advance and reviewed at the campsite. See activity checkpoints on Cooking, Food Preparation, and Cleaning and Cooking Fires.

Rafting

(Also refer to Boating activity checkpoints.)

Planning and Supervision

❏ At least one adult guide with documented experience indicating knowledge and skill in teaching and/or supervising rafting must oversee the activity.

❏ The guides must know the International Scale of River Difficulty and the Universal River Signals from the American Whitewater Affiliation and its Safety Code.

❏ One adult must be trained and experienced in river rescue techniques.

❏ A minimum of two adults must supervise any rafting activity.

❏ All girls' comfort level in the water must be assessed, as described in the Boating activity checkpoints on page 70, in order to go rafting.

❏ All rafters must receive prior instruction in how to float through rapids, how to breathe while swimming in rapids, and how to swim to shore.

❏ All participants must be trained in rescue and recovery skills appropriate to the raft and the site.

Clothing

❏ Laced sneakers or other nonslip footwear designed for water sports must be worn on shore and in the raft.

❏ For protection against hypothermia, a wetsuit must be worn when the water temperature is below 50°F. When the combined air and water temperature is less than 100°F or when the combination of cool air, wind chill, and evaporative cooling may lead to hypothermia, a wetsuit should be worn.

❏ Dressing in layers—using wool, nylon, or polypropylene pile under a jacket and pants made of coated materials to repel water—will help to protect the body from getting chilled.

Equipment

❏ Each raft must be of heavy-duty construction, have four or more air compartments, an adequate number of large D-rings securely attached to the sides, and snug hand lines along the sides.

❏ Rafts should be in good repair and appropriate to the trip.

❏ A PFD must be worn by each participant.

❏ A safety helmet must be worn when rafting in Class III and above waters.

❏ The safety helmet must be a properly fitted, flexible, plastic shell with a chin strap and openings for drainage.

❏ Throw lines, throw bags, a repair kit, emergency kit, knives, whistles, bailers, and foot pump must be carried on the rafting trip.

Site

❏ Council guidance must be obtained in selecting rafting sites.

❏ No trip shall be taken on water that has not been run and rated. No trip shall be taken on whitewater more difficult than Class IV as defined by the American Version of the International Version of River Difficulty.

Emergency Procedures and First Aid

❑ One adult must have current first-aid training.

❑ A first-aid kit must be kept within reach of the first-aider. The kit must be in a waterproof container and secured in the raft.

❑ First-aid procedures must be reviewed, including those for immersion hypothermia, near-drowning, sprains, and fractures.

❑ Arrangements must be made in advance for medical emergencies and evacuation procedures.

National Organizations

American Canoe Association, America Outdoors, National Organization for River Sports.

Roller Skating

Asterisks to the left of boxes on this page indicate items that also apply to Outdoor Roller Skating on page 98.

Planning and Supervision

Roller Skating Rink:

*❑ All girls must receive basic instruction in roller skating skills.

❑ Leaders must supervise from outside the main skating floor. (Check with the rink manager in advance to learn how many adults, in addition to the rink staff, are needed to supervise the group.)

❑ Practice sessions must be scheduled for beginners.

❑ The rink manager must be called in advance to arrange for large groups or for practice sessions.

❑ The rink must be adequately staffed to monitor and control the behavior and the size of the crowd.

*❑ Girls must learn to perform basic roller skating skills before attempting more advanced skills.

*❑ Girls must learn how to fall and get up correctly as a beginning skill.

*❑ Warm-up exercises must be done before any strenuous roller skating; cool-down exercises must end the sessions.

*❑ Roller skaters must be instructed on safety rules by the leader or rink manager or both.

❑ The rules of the rink must be observed.

For example:

❑ Everyone must skate in the same direction.

❑ Girls should not stop in the main roller skating area.

❑ Skaters must yield the right-of-way to those already in the rink.

❑ Skaters must not cut across the paths of other skaters.

❏ Skaters must not push, shove, or race.

❏ A falling roller skater must not grab hold of another skater.

❏ A fallen skater must rise quickly, unless injured.

❏ Loose or sharp articles, such as handbags, combs, keys, etc., must not be carried in pockets, hands, hair, or anyplace where they might fall to the floor or injure a falling skater.

Outdoor Roller Skating:

❏ Refer to all starred items in the "Roller Skating Rink" section on page 97.

❏ Girls must never roller-skate in the street or in a parking lot that is being used.

❏ Girls must skate in areas where traffic or pedestrians will not interfere. Check local ordinances for any restrictions.

❏ Girls must not skate faster than their ability to stop.

❏ Girls must not roller-skate alone or at night.

❏ Girls must use the buddy system.

❏ Roller skaters must be alert to their surroundings.

❏ Girls must not wear headphones while roller skating.

Clothing

❏ Clothing must allow freedom of movement.

Equipment

❏ Girls must receive instruction in selecting the proper skate size.

❏ Roller skates must be properly fitted, securely laced, and properly tied.

❏ Roller skate wheels, boots, and plates must be kept in good condition and inspected. The wheels must be kept clean and checked for wear.

❏ Never skate with broken or missing laces. Dangling decorations must not be attached to laces.

❏ When roller skating outdoors, protective gear must include elbow pads and kneepads, wrist guards, and a helmet with the American National Standards Institute (ANSI) or SNELL Memorial Foundation seal or both.

Site

❏ Council guidance must be obtained in selecting the roller skating site. Roller skating rinks are the safest places to skate.

Roller Skating Rink:

❏ A rink must have a smooth skating surface free from papers, candy wrappers, and other debris.

❏ The rink safety rules must be posted or announced or both, and practiced.

Outdoor Roller Skating:

❏ Skating surfaces must be checked in advance for cracks, uneven joints and grooves, twigs, pebbles, or bits of glass that might cause a fall.

Local ordinances or parks offices must be checked to see if roller skating is permitted on bike paths or in city parks.

Additional Checkpoints for In-Line Roller Skates

❏ Beginners must receive instruction.

❏ Beginners must use four-wheel in-line skates.

❏ Skates must be equipped with a brake.

❏ Protective equipment, including helmets, kneepads, elbow pads, and wrist pads must be worn.

❏ In-line skating helmets or bicycle helmets that carry the SNELL Memorial Foundation or American National Standards Institute (ANSI) seal must be worn. The seal is usually on the inside of the helmet.

Emergency Prodedures and First Aid

Roller Skating Rink:

❏ A first-aid kit must be available.

Outdoor Roller Skating:

❏ An adult with current first-aid training must be present.

❏ A first-aid kit must be available.

National Organizations

Roller Skating Rink Operators Association, United States Amateur Confederation of Roller Skating.

Rowboating

(Also refer to Boating activity checkpoints.)

Planning and Supervision

❏ One adult must have certification in Small Craft Safety from the American Red Cross or experience in teaching and/or supervising rowboating.

❏ The instructor/qualified leader to participant ratio for rowboating is 1–12.

❏ A minimum of two adults must supervise any rowboating activity.

❏ On a controlled waterfront, a checkboard system must be used to determine the number and location of rowboaters.

❏ Each girl's comfort level in the water must be assessed, as described in the Boating activity checkpoint on page 70, in order to go rowboating.

Clothing

❏ Laced sneakers or other nonslip footwear designed for water sports must be worn while rowing.

❏ A hat and sunscreen should be worn, if appropriate.

Equipment

❏ Each person must wear a PFD.

❏ Rowboats must have painters (also called end or grab lines) secured to each end of the boat. The bow painter must be made of strong line that floats and is approximately the length of the rowboat.

❏ Oars must be in good repair and sized and balanced for the rowboat.

❏ A bailer must be in each rowboat.

❏ Rowboat weight and capacity must not be exceeded.

Site

❏ Council guidance must be obtained in selecting a rowboating site.

❏ Marine and weather forecasts must be obtained and monitored for the area where the boating will take place.

Emergency Procedures and First Aid

❏ One adult with current first-aid training must be present.

❏ A first-aid kit must be available.

❏ First-aid procedures must be reviewed, including those for immersion hypothermia, near-drowning, and sunburn.

❏ In case of injury, arrangements must be made in advance for medical emergencies and evacuation procedures.

❏ In the event of an electrical storm, if shore cannot be reached, secure all loose gear, keep a sharp lookout for other boats and obstructions, head into the wind at a 45° angle, and stay low.

National Organization

American Red Cross, U.S. Rowing Association.

Sailing

(Also refer to Boating activity checkpoints.)

Planning and Supervision

❏ One adult must be currently certified as a Sailing Instructor by the U.S. Sailing Association (formerly U.S. Yacht Racing Union—USYRU), or Small Craft Safety certification from the American Red Cross, or have equivalent certification or documented experience and skill in teaching and/or supervising sailing.

❏ A minimum of two adults must supervise any sailing activity. The number of persons who supervise sailing must be determined by the skill level of the sailors, degree of risk, and environmental conditions.

❏ All girls' comfort level in the water must be assessed, as described in the Boating activity checkpoints on page 70, in order to go sailing.

❏ Instruction must include launching safety and line handling.

❏ All participants must be instructed in the care and use of ropes, including knot tying and splicing.

❏ The techniques and skills of anchoring the craft must be practiced. Special attention must be paid to anchoring in restricted water.

❏ A motorized chase boat must be available for all sailing activities, where conditions permit.

❏ Girls must be trained in self-rescue procedures in case the wind stops blowing or they are in an emergency situation.

❏ Rules set up by the U.S. Sailing Association must be followed for sail racing.

Clothing

❏ Laced sneakers or other nonslip footwear designed for water sports must be worn.

❏ When appropriate, girls must wear a hat and sunglasses and use sunscreen.

Equipment

❏ A PFD must be worn by each participant.

❏ Each sailboat must be in good repair.

❏ There must be a repair kit available that is equipped with items such as a screwdriver, pliers, shackles, extra line, a sewing kit, and electrical tape for on-the-water repairs.

❏ A paddle must be in each sailboat to provide a second means of propulsion.

Site

❏ Council guidance must be obtained in selecting sailing sites.

❏ An area for mooring and dock-landing practice must be provided that is away from other aquatic activities.

❏ The launching area must be clear of overhead power lines.

❏ The weather conditions must be known and suitable before going sailing, and they must be monitored during the trip.

Emergency Procedures and First Aid

❏ An adult with current first-aid training must be present.

❏ A first-aid kit must be available.

❏ First-aid procedures must be reviewed, including those for immersion hypothermia, near-drowning, and sunburn.

❏ In a calm-water situation, all participants must be instructed in and practice the procedures for dealing with sailing emergencies, such as running aground, person overboard, etc.

❏ Arrangements must be made in advance for medical emergencies and evacuation procedures.

National Organizations

American Red Cross, American Sail Training Association, U.S. Sailing Association (formerly U.S. Yacht Racing Union—USYRU).

Science-Related Activities

Planning and Supervision

❏ When any specialized equipment or chemicals are used, one adult with experience and knowledge must be present to teach skills and demonstrate the use of the equipment.

❏ The instructor must be responsible for the safe use and proper care of all equipment and materials.

❏ Science activities taken from the Girl Scout handbooks and related resources should be done as outlined in the materials.

❏ The activity must be appropriate for each girl's age, experience, and expertise.

❏ All outdoor science activities, such as field investigations, night hikes, astronomy lessons, cave explorations, or stream studies, must be carried out with the proper supervision of the girls.

Equipment and Materials

❏ The work area must be ample and appropriate for the science activity.

When working with any chemical, plant, or animal, the following must be observed:

❏ Hands must not touch the mouth or face during the activity.

❏ Facilities for washing hands and eyes must be available at the site.

❏ Hands must be washed thoroughly after the activity.

❏ The equipment must be thoroughly cleaned.

❏ Used materials must be disposed of in a proper manner.

❏ Chemical substances must be used or mixed only when the instructor specifically knows the outcome. When chemicals are used, goggles stamped ANSI Z87 on the frame and lens must be worn. Even the simplest experiment can be an eye hazard.

Plants

In showing concern for the environment, accepted practice is not to pick any plant species unless there is a real need. Most observations can be carried out while the plant is in its natural surroundings.

❑ If it is necessary to pick a plant, the instructor must be familiar with the species and the possible allergic reactions or chemical sensitivity that may be caused by handling the plant.

❑ Girls must wash their hands after handling seeds.

❑ Seeds must not be placed in the mouth, as they may be coated with insecticides, fungicides, or other chemicals.

Animals

Activities done with animals must be carried out with sensitivity and concern for the needs of the animals.

❑ Aquariums and terrariums must be kept in areas where proper care, temperature regulation, and maintenance are always possible.

❑ Girls must be aware of the proper care, feeding, and maintenance of the animals, and take appropriate

responsibility for meeting these needs.

Site

❑ There must be sufficient space to move around while working.

❑ There must be well-ventilated areas for the use of vaporous materials such as chemicals.

❑ Flammable materials must be kept in fireproof containers and in an area away from ignition sources.

❑ Food or beverages must not be consumed in an activity area. Hands must be washed before eating.

❑ A fire extinguisher must be available when flammable materials are used.

Emergency Procedures and First Aid

❑ An adult with current first-aid training must be present.

❑ A first-aid kit must be readily available and first-aid procedures must be known and practiced regularly.

❑ Medical care must be easily accessible.

National Organizations

Association for Women in Science, National Safety Council, National Science Teachers Association.

Skiing (Cross-Country)

Planning and Supervision

❑ Instruction must be given by an adult with experience in teaching and/or supervising cross-country skiing for the age group(s) involved.

❑ At least four people must be in the cross-country skiing group, including a minimum of two adults.

❑ An adult must lead. Another adult must bring up the rear of the skiing group.

❑ Girls must get in condition by exercising prior to skiing.

❑ Leaders must be aware of each girl's ability.

❑ Practice sessions must be scheduled for beginners.

The rules of the cross-country ski area must be explained and observed:

❑ Girls must ski under control to avoid other skiers and objects.

❑ Girls must yield the right-of-way to those already on the trail. They must step to the side to let other skiers pass. A descending skier has the right of way.

❑ A faster skier must indicate her desire to pass by calling "Track, please."

❑ Girls must not ski close to the edge of an embankment or cliff.

❑ Girls must not walk on ski trails.

❑ Sitzmarks (crash craters) must be filled in.

Clothing

❑ Protective clothing appropriate for the weather must be worn.

❑ Hats, gloves or mittens, and heavy insulating socks should be worn.

❑ A windproof, waterproof parka or jacket should be worn.

Equipment

❑ Girls must use equipment that fits properly and is in good working order.

❑ All equipment must be inspected before use.

❑ Sunglasses or goggles must be worn to protect the eyes from the bright glare of the snow.

❑ Each girl must carry water, high-energy food, sunscreen, and lip balm.

Transportation

❑ Transportation plans must be made in advance and confirmed before departure.

Site

❑ Council approval must be obtained in selecting the site.

At the trail:

☐ Safety rules must be reviewed.

☐ The route chosen must be within the ability of every girl in the group.

☐ The nature of the terrain, potential hazards (e.g., avalanches, frozen lakes), mileage, and approximate cross-country skiing time must be known to all members of the group.

☐ The weather conditions must be suitable and monitored.

☐ There must be adequate rest stops with an opportunity to replenish fluids and to eat high-energy foods.

☐ If applicable, a fire-building permit or permission to camp must be obtained (see activity checkpoints for Cooking Fires and Troop Camping).

☐ Respect for wildlife and the environment must be demonstrated.

☐ Girls must have training in winter survival (e.g., snow cave building, whiteouts, avalanche avoidance, etc.) as needed.

Emergency Procedures and First Aid

☐ An adult with current first-aid training must be present.

☐ A first-aid kit must be available.

☐ First-aid procedures must be reviewed, including those for frostbite, cold exposure, hypothermia, sprains, fractures, and altitude sickness.

☐ The itinerary, with planned departure and return times and names of the cross-country skiers, must be left with a contact person. The route must be marked on a map. Before starting out and upon return, the contact person must be advised.

☐ Security plans and procedures must be established.

☐ Search-and-rescue procedures must be written out in advance.

☐ Arrangements must be made in advance for medical emergencies and evacuation procedures.

National Organization

National Ski Patrol.

Skiing (Downhill)

These checkpoints can also be applied to snowboarding.

Planning and Supervision

☐ Consult with your council for guidance and approval.

☐ Instruction must be given by a person with experience in teaching and/or supervising downhill skiing for the age group(s) involved.

☐ Participants must condition themselves by exercising prior to the trip.

❑ Leaders must be aware of each girl's ability.

❑ Lessons and practice sessions must be scheduled for beginners and conducted by qualified instructors.

❑ All skiers must receive instruction on how to ride area lifts, including line courtesy, loading and unloading, and emergency procedures.

❑ All skiers must ski responsibly. The rules pertaining to the downhill ski area must be explained and observed.

❑ Skiers must use the buddy system and must ski on trails and slopes matched to their abilities. At all times, skiers must ski under control. These guidelines must be followed:

❑ Avoid other skiers.

❑ Avoid objects and obstacles.

❑ Make other skiers aware that you are planning turns.

❑ Do not cross the path of other uphill skiers.

❑ Yield the right-of-way to those already on the slope.

❑ Stop on the sides of the slope or trail when resting or adjusting equipment.

❑ Summon the ski patrol in case of injury to a skier.

❑ Move quickly to the side of the trail or slope after falling, unless injured.

❑ Never ski in unmarked or closed areas.

❑ There must be adequate rest periods that include an opportunity to replenish fluids and eat high-energy foods.

❑ A nutritious, high-energy menu must be planned, with beverages provided to combat dehydration.

Clothing

❑ Protective clothing appropriate for the weather must be worn.

❑ Hats, gloves or mittens, and heavy insulating socks should be worn.

❑ A windproof, waterproof parka or jacket should be worn.

Equipment

❑ Girls must use equipment that fits properly, is appropriate to their skill level, and is in good working order.

❑ All equipment must be inspected before use and bindings adjusted to each individual skier.

❑ Girls must receive proper instruction on use of equipment and safety features.

❑ Sunglasses or goggles must be worn to protect the eyes from the bright glare of snow.

Transportation

❑ Transportation arrangements should be made in advance and confirmed before departure.

Site

❏ Council approval must be obtained in selecting the site.

At the slope:

❏ A list must be maintained of each skier and where she plans to ski.

❏ Safety rules must be reviewed.

❏ There must be at least two in each skiing party.

❏ The slope chosen must be within the ability of each girl in the skiing party.

❏ Terrain and potential hazards must be known to each girl in the group.

❏ Weather conditions must be suitable and monitored.

❏ A designated meeting place must be established where girls can contact an adult in charge of the group.

Emergency Procedures and First Aid

❏ An adult with current first-aid training must be present.

❏ A first-aid kit must be available.

❏ First-aid procedures must be reviewed, including those for frostbite, cold exposure, hypothermia, sprains, and fractures.

❏ Arrangements must be made in advance for medical emergencies and evacuation procedures.

National Organization

National Ski Patrol.

Sports

Planning and Supervision

❏ Council advice must be obtained on the safety, inherent risks, and appropriateness of the sport.

❏ Instruction must be given by an adult who has experience, knowledge, and skill in teaching and/or supervision specific to the sport being played.

❏ Where necessary, trained officials must administer the rules of the sport.

❏ Girls must be provided with adequate conditioning and with practice in basic skills.

❏ Warm-up and cool-down exercises and stretching techniques must be conducted to reduce the incidence of sprains, strains, and other injuries.

❏ In competition, girls must be matched in age, weight, height, skill, and physical maturation.

❏ Girls must be aware of their capabilities and limitations.

❏ In team sports, positions and sides must be rotated to prevent domination of the game and to allow for full participation.

❑ Trained spotters and/or instructors' assistants must be used for individual sports such as gymnastics.

❑ Practice sessions and games should be properly supervised and reasonable in length.

❑ Practice or competition may only occur when an instructor and/or supervisor is present at the site of play.

❑ Sufficient rest periods must be given to avoid overexertion and to replenish fluid intake.

Clothing

❑ Girls must wear comfortable, protective clothing and footwear that is appropriate for the activity.

❑ Loose articles, such as jewelry or combs, must not be worn or carried in pockets. Pierced earrings must be removed.

Equipment

❑ Girls must wear quality protective equipment that is in good condition.

❑ All equipment must be inspected before use and a maintenance check done periodically. Records of maintenance checks, requests, and repairs must be kept for the life of the equipment.

❑ Where necessary, equipment and rules must be adapted to meet the developmental levels of the girls.

❑ There must be sufficient floor mats for gymnastics, tumbling, and similar activities.

❑ Girls who wear glasses must have shatterproof lenses or wear glass guards. A band should be worn to hold glasses securely.

Transportation

❑ Transportation arrangements must be made in advance and plans confirmed before departure.

Site

❑ Council guidance must be obtained in selecting appropriate sports facilities, such as a gymnasium.

❑ There must be periodic safety and maintenance checks of facilities. Records of maintenance checks, requests, and repairs must be kept.

❑ Playing surfaces must be smooth and clear of obstructions, broken glass, etc.

❑ Playing areas must have clearly marked boundaries and adequate space for girls to move around freely.

❑ Where necessary, there should be adequate protection for spectators.

❑ The weather conditions must be suitable and monitored.

❑ Outdoor activity must be suspended during an electrical storm or in very hot, humid weather.

❑ There must be ample, safe drinking water available.

Emergency Procedures and First-Aid

☐ Proper medical care must be easily accessible.

☐ One adult must have current first-aid training.

☐ A first-aid kit must be available.

☐ Fatigued or injured girls must be removed from competition and cared for promptly.

☐ In case of serious injury, a girl must not be moved until trained emergency medical service personnel arrive. An injured girl must not be returned to practice or competition without the approval of a physician.

National Organizations

American Alliance for Health, Physical Education, Recreation, and Dance; National Association for Girls and Women in Sports.

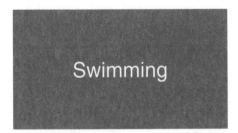

Swimming

Planning and Supervision

Use the following chart to determine the number of lifeguards and watchers needed for swimming activities.

Swimming Activities in pools, lakes, slow-moving streams, and rivers:

Lifeguard-Watcher Ratio Chart		
Number of Swimmers	Lifeguards	Watchers
1–10	1+	1*
11–25	1+	2*
26–35	2+*	3*
36–50	2+*	4*

+ Primary lifeguard must be an adult.

* May be a person who is under the age of majority for the state in which the activity will take place, but cannot be under 16 years of age.

Note: At no time can the number of lifeguards and watchers under the age of majority be greater than the number of adult lifeguards and watchers. For swimming in backyard pools, use one lifeguard for 1–10 swimmers. The lifeguard must be a minimum of 16 years old, with certification in Lifeguard Training or equivalent. An adult trained in water rescue skills must also be present. American Red Cross Basic Water Rescue is recommended.

Swimming Activities in oceans, large bays, and wide, rapidly running rivers.

One currently certified adult lifeguard plus one watcher is on duty for every 10 swimmers.

Wading. When girls are wading in water more than knee-deep, an adult with American Red Cross Basic Water Rescue certification, or with documented experience in basic water rescue skills, must be present. A ratio of one watcher to 10 girls must be maintained.

The following apply to all swimming activities:

☐ When on duty, the lifeguards and watchers must stay out of the water except in emergencies.

❑ Lifeguards and watchers must be stationed at separate posts.

❑ Each participant must be tested and classified according to her swimming ability. Untested participants must be limited to shallow water.

❑ Public pools and controlled waterfronts may be used when lifeguards are on duty in ratios designed by the facility operator.

❑ In crowded areas, a color system must be used for identification. Nonswimmers, novice swimmers, and skilled swimmers must each have a wrist band or hair band of a different color.

❑ In a controlled waterfront, a checkboard system must be used, indicating which girls are in the water and in which swimming area.

❑ The buddy system must be used.

❑ The length of a swimming period must be determined by the swimmer's condition and comfort, the weather conditions, and the water temperature. Generally, 30-minute swimming periods are sufficient.

❑ Instruction must be given in basic swimming rules:

> ❑ Girls must not dive into aboveground pools, shallow areas, etc.
>
> ❑ Girls must swim in supervised areas only.
>
> ❑ Girls must not swim immediately after eating, when overheated, or when tired.
>
> ❑ Girls must swim at a safe distance from any diving board.
>
> ❑ Girls must swim with a buddy.

❑ Girls must learn and practice proper use of personal flotation devices (PFDs) and other rescue equipment.

Equipment

❑ Basic rescue equipment must be immediately available:

> ❑ Reaching pole approximately 12 feet long (or appropriate to the site)
>
> ❑ Ring buoy or throw bag with firmly attached line approximately 30 feet long
>
> ❑ Rescue tube
>
> ❑ Backboard

❑ Electrical appliances, such as radios or portable telephones, must not be used in or near swimming areas.

Site

Whether using council-owned or -operated swimming sites, or public, loaned, or donated facilities, the same general principles must be observed in every situation:

❑ Girl Scout council guidance must be obtained in selecting a site. Public pools, supervised beaches, and other waterfront areas that provide instruction and lifeguards are usually the safest places.

❑ At public facilities, the water quality must pass the local health department tests. Where needed, obtain a copy of the report from the local health department or use a pool test kit.

❏ Bottles, glass, and other sharp objects must not be allowed in the swimming area.

❏ Swimming ability areas must be clearly defined.

❏ Girls may swim only during daylight hours or in a well-lit pool at night.

❏ The weather and water conditions must be suitable for the activity. Consider wind, waves, water and air temperature, electrical storms, etc.

❏ In the event of an electrical storm, swimmers must leave the water immediately, move away from the water, seek low ground and shelter, and must not stand under a prominent tree.

❏ Safety rules must be understood, practiced, and posted.

❏ An emergency telephone must be available, whenever possible.

Swimming Pool

❏ Local and state ordinances should be observed.

❏ Local health department pool sanitation regulations must be observed.

❏ The pool water depths must be clearly marked.

❏ Shallow areas must be marked "No Diving."

❏ There must be periodic maintenance checks. Records of maintenance requests and repairs must be documented and retained.

❏ The water pH and chlorine levels must be tested and maintained at safe levels. Records of tests must be documented and retained.

❏ The pool must be adequately filtered so that the water is clear.

❏ The decks around the pool must be kept clean and free of clutter.

❏ The surrounding fence and gate or doors to the pool must be locked when the pool is not being supervised.

Beach or Other Waterfront Area

❏ Hazards must be eliminated or clearly marked.

❏ Girls must be instructed to avoid strong currents, sharp drop-offs, quicksand bottoms, rough surf, and other potentially dangerous conditions.

❏ As best as can be determined, the water must be free from dangerous marine life.

❏ The bottom must be relatively free from debris, sharp stones, and shells.

❏ Diving and boating areas must be separate. They must be clearly marked or roped off or both.

Sliding Boards

☐ Only one person may be on the slide at a time.

☐ Girls must slide in a sitting position, never headfirst.

☐ The landing area must be off-limits to other swimmers.

☐ The landing area must be cleared before the next slider starts.

☐ The water depth in the slide landing area must be at least five feet deep.

Diving Areas

☐ The diving area must be divided from the swimming area by a buoyed line.

☐ There must be a minimum water depth of 12 feet in the landing area for safe diving from competitive diving boards. They are usually 16 feet long and 3 to 10 feet above the water's surface.

☐ There must be a minimum depth of 10 feet in the landing area for safe diving from recreational diving boards. They are usually 12 to 14 feet long and less than 3 feet above the water's surface.

☐ Diving must be restricted to water of sufficient depth and checked in advance for submerged obstructions. Diving is prohibited in waters where depth and conditions are not known.

☐ Recreational divers must not manipulate the adjustable fulcrum on springboards. During recreational swimming periods, the adjustable fulcrum must be locked in a fixed position, preferably in its most forward position, in order to reduce the spring of the board.

☐ The maximum water depth must extend laterally 10 feet on either side from the center line of the board. The water depth is subject to change by the effect of tides, drought, and similar forces, and must be checked each time before diving is permitted.

☐ Girls must not dive off the side of the board.

Emergency Procedures and First Aid

☐ An adult with current first-aid training must be present.

☐ The first-aider must be prepared to handle cases of near-drowning, immersion hypothermia, and sunburn.

☐ A first-aid kit must be available.

☐ A list of emergency telephone numbers, including nearby physician, ambulance, hospital, police, and fire or rescue unit, must be posted.

☐ All girls must know self-help techniques for emergencies, such as cramps.

☐ All girls must know and practice basic rescue techniques, such as reaching with a hand or towel, throwing a ring buoy or throw bag, extending a kick board, etc.

❑ The procedures to follow in case of a lost swimmer or other emergency must be written down, reviewed, and practiced.

❑ In the event of an electrical storm, move away from the water, and seek low ground and shelter. If a sheltered area is not available, crouch low to the ground in an open area. Stay away from tall, solitary objects, such as trees or electrical poles.

National Organization

American Red Cross, United States Swimming, Inc.

Theme Park Activities

Planning and Supervision

❑ Girls must be accompanied by adults in the appropriate ratios. (See Program Standard 13, Guideline B.)

❑ Adults must check in advance to make sure that the park carries liability insurance.

❑ In the planning stages, adults must obtain full information about the rides and other activities and evaluate them in terms of safety. The park manager or safety officer should be willing to discuss safety,

maintenance programs, insurance coverage, or other matters of concern.

❑ Each girl must be instructed to consider her own personal limitations with regard to rides. How is she affected by height, speed, movement, etc.? Theme parks have policies and signage restricting access to certain rides because of height, weight, or other criteria.

❑ Leaders must instruct girls to look for and comply with all park safety-related signs and instructions given by ride operators.

Clothing

❑ Casual and comfortable clothing suitable for the weather must be worn. On sunny or hazy days, protection from the sun will be needed.

❑ All hats, glasses, purses, and other such items must be secured during the ride or not taken on the ride.

❑ Long, flowing garments and dangling jewelry may be a problem on some rides and must not be worn.

❑ Girls must wear comfortable walking shoes that provide good traction.

Site

❑ The adult leaders must determine the appropriate time of day and length of the visit to the theme park.

❑ Upon arrival, a copy of the park guide must be obtained. This will facilitate the visit, and will provide important information on park policies and the location of restrooms and the first-aid station. Special attention must be paid to any safety tips or warnings. This information must be shared with the girls.

☐ Leaders and girls must discuss a "lost plan" and set a place to meet in case of separation from the adult in charge or from the group.

☐ Girls must obey signs concerning age/height/weight restrictions on rides, listen to the instructions from ride operators, and note the location of ride exits and emergency routes.

☐ In extremely hot weather, it is advisable to go on rides and do other outdoor activities in the morning and late afternoon hours, and to go inside for meals, stage shows, etc., during the warmest time of the day.

☐ On rides, girls and adults must remain seated at all times and must always keep their arms and legs inside the car.

☐ Seat belts or restraint bars must always be used and **never** removed during rides.

☐ Any unsafe conditions, such as slippery floors, broken seat belts, nonfunctioning exit signs, etc., must be reported to the nearest park attendant.

Emergency Procedures and First Aid

☐ In the event of illness or accident, the nearest park attendant must be notified.

☐ Medical care must be easily accessible.

☐ First-aid equipment and supplies should be readily available, and first-aid procedures should be known and practiced.

National Organization

International Association of Amusement Parks and Attractions

Trip/Travel Camping

Trip camping is planned and carried out by a group of girls who are experienced campers and adult leaders. The group camps at different sites for three or more nights and travels from one site to another under its own power or by transportation that permits individual guidance of the vehicle or animal (for example, bicycle, canoe, horse, sailboat).

Travel camping (using campsites as a means of accommodation) or traveling groups (using other than campsites as a means of accommodation) are planned and carried out by a group of girls who are experienced campers and by adult leadership. The group uses motorized transportation to move from one site to another over a period of three or more nights. Motorized transportation is normally a bus, van, or automobile, but it may also include an airplane, boat, train, or a combination of these vehicles.

Planning and Supervision

Activity checkpoints in this book should be used in preparing for and conducting the trip, depending on the mode of travel (canoeing, backpacking, kayaking, bicycling, skiing) and/or activities engaged in, such as cooking or swimming.

❑ The trip/travel camping leader must possess knowledge, skills, and experience in the following areas:

   ❑ Outdoor leadership
   ❑ Progression and readiness
   ❑ Trip planning
   ❑ Minimal-impact camping
   ❑ Safety management
   ❑ First aid, safety, handling of emergency situations
   ❑ Judgment and maturity
   ❑ Program activities specific to the trip
   ❑ Group dynamics and management
   ❑ Supervision of both campers and staff
   ❑ Participation in similar trips
   ❑ Familiarity with the area in which the trip is conducted
   ❑ Physical fitness and skills necessary to lead the group

❑ A minimum of two adult leaders must be present on each trip. In addition, the adult to girl ratio as set in Program Standard 13 and/or in the specific activity checkpoint or mode of travel involved must be followed.

❑ Adult leaders selected for the trip must be trained or have documented experience in the following areas:

   ❑ Travel or trip camping skills
   ❑ Minimal-impact camping skills
   ❑ Group management and group dynamics
   ❑ Child development
   ❑ Mode of transportation
   ❑ Site orientation
   ❑ First aid and cardiopulmonary resuscitation
   ❑ Emergency procedures
   ❑ Operational procedures
   ❑ Minor maintenance for equipment and vehicle, as appropriate

❑ At least one adult leader on each trip must be currently trained in first aid.

A pretrip/pretravel orientation must be given for each trip that involves girls and leaders and includes the following:

   ❑ First-aid procedures
   ❑ Emergency and rescue procedures
   ❑ Environmental awareness and protection procedures
   ❑ Program plans related to mode of travel and geographic area

❏ Operational procedures
1 Purification of water
2 Food preparation
3 Camp equipment
4 Sanitation procedures
5 Food storage procedures

❏ If aquatic activities occur on the trip, a person with the following qualifications supervises the aquatic activities. For aquatic trips, an adult who:

❏ Is currently certified in lifeguarding or who has taken training in river rescue, small-craft rescue, or the equivalent, as appropriate.

❏ Has an instructor rating in the appropriate craft or documented experience in that type of trip.

For other trips:

❏ An adult who is currently certified in lifeguarding or the equivalent.

❏ There must be a currently signed agreement with providers of trip/travel camping services that specifies responsibility for compliance with these trip/travel camping guidelines.

Clothing

❏ Clothing suitable for the weather and terrain must be worn.

Equipment

❏ Only suitable camping equipment in good working order may be used. Girls and adult leaders should be protected from the natural elements (rain, snow, wind, sun, cold, insects, ticks, etc.) by the following, as appropriate to geographic location and season:

❏ Shelter
❏ Clothing
❏ Sleeping gear
❏ Repellents
❏ Sun blocks

❏ All girls and leaders must wear an identifying bracelet or similar device with the following information on it:

❏ Name of girl or adult
❏ Name of Girl Scout council
❏ Telephone number for emergency contact

❏ In addition, all girls and adult leaders participating in a trip must have on their person a card with their name, address, and telephone number; the council name, address, and telephone number; and the name of a contact person.

Transportation

❏ Each driver of motorized transportation must be at least 21 years old and hold a valid operator's license appropriate to the vehicle. The operator's driving record must be checked.

❏ There must be a relief driver for trips of more than four hours. The relief driver must hold a valid operator's license for the vehicle operated, and her/his driving record must be checked.

❏ If a trailer is used, it must be in compliance with all state, local, and federal regulations for the areas of travel. The staff assigned to drive will be experienced in pulling a trailer. No girls or adult leaders will ride in the trailer.

Site

❏ All permissions required (camping, hiking, fire permit, etc.) for all travel sites and the necessary permissions or reservations must be obtained prior to the use of the site(s). The trip/travel leaders should be aware of the procedures required by those permits/permissions.

❏ Written procedures should be in practice for conducting each trip with minimal environmental impact, including procedures regarding (where appropriate):

  ❏ Group limits—based upon the environmental carrying capacity of the site(s). Limits do not exceed those set by other jurisdictional authorities.

  ❏ Refuse disposal—requirement that all refuse be carried out or disposed of in accordance with regulations governing each area.

❏ Soap—only biodegradable and nondetergent soap is used at campsites, unless medically advised otherwise.

❏ Human waste disposal sites—located a minimum of 200 feet from any water supply, trail, or campsite. Human waste should be disposed of in a manner that accelerates decomposition.

❏ Site selection—use an established, well-worn site rather than start a new one. Leave few signs of your use.

Emergency Procedures and First Aid

❏ A written itinerary should be filed with the council office and with jurisdictional authorities (when they are available and will accept itineraries).

❏ There must be written procedures to follow should a person (leader or girl) need to be removed from the trip.

❏ A communication system regarding progress of the trip should be maintained between the trip group and the council office.

❏ Medical assistance and phone numbers for an emergency on the trip and a record of the exact locations of medical assistance and phone numbers for emergency help must be carried on the trip. A completed copy of the trip plan must be on file with the council office.

Troop Camping

Planning and Supervision

☐ The leader must have taken council troop camp training in teaching and supervising troop camping. As an alternative, a program consultant trained in troop camping may help the leader and the girls prepare for the troop camping trip and then accompany the leader and troop on the trip.

☐ Troop camp training generally must cover these topics:

  ☐ Girl Scout program activities appropriate to the outdoor setting

  ☐ The use of troop government in a camp setting

  ☐ Group preparation for the trip

  ☐ Resources of the site and surrounding area

  ☐ Activities and camping skills that represent steps in progression

  ☐ Safety standards, activity checkpoints, and council policies for camping and outdoor activities

  ☐ Procedures for cookouts, kapers, and special activities

  ☐ Minimal-impact camping skills

  ☐ First-aid and other emergency procedures

  ☐ Methods of dealing with homesickness

  ☐ Awareness and understanding of differing social, economic, and ethnic backgrounds

  ☐ Discussion of other camping opportunities available to troop members, including day, core-staff, and resident camp, and wider opportunities

☐ Each troop must be accompanied by a minimum of two adults. The girl/leader ratios given in Program Standard 13 must be observed.

☐ The size of the group should be planned to minimize the group's impact on the campsite and the environment.

☐ The type of facilities used, the duration of the trip, and the activities planned must be determined by the needs and interests of the girls, their physical and emotional readiness, and their experience and skill level.

☐ Girls must participate in the planning and preparation for the trip. Girls plan menus, activities, rules for group living, and on-site activities.

☐ Girls must learn about appropriate clothing, footwear, bedding, packing, personal health care, and ways to dress for changes in weather conditions.

☐ Girls must be adequately instructed and prepared for the planned activities.

☐ Safety rules must be observed for cooking, fire building, portable stove use, hiking, swimming, science activities, boating, etc. (Refer to the appropriate activity checkpoints for further information on these topics.)

Clothing

❑ Clothing suitable for the weather and terrain must be worn.

❑ Shoes or tennis shoes and socks must always be worn; no sandals, flip-flops, or bare feet.

Equipment

❑ Only suitable camping equipment in good working order may be used.

❑ Sleeping bags must be stuffed with filler appropriate for the anticipated temperature (check the label).

❑ Candles, kerosene lamps, portable cookstoves, or anything with an open flame must **never** be used inside tents. Battery-powered lights are recommended. Lanterns fueled by propane, butane, kerosene, or gasoline may be used out-of-doors.

❑ Heaters may not be used inside tents.

❑ All tents must be made of flame-retardant, fiber-impregnated materials. Plastic tents may not be used.

❑ Food must never be stored inside sleeping tents.

Transportation

❑ Transportation arrangements must be made in advance. Plans must be confirmed before departure. Safety procedures must be reviewed with the driver and passengers.

Site

❑ Council approval must be obtained.

❑ State and local regulations related to drinking water, sanitation, fire building, etc., must be observed.

❑ The site must be inspected or a firsthand report obtained in advance to assess any hazards and the suitability of the site for the troop.

❑ Potentially dangerous areas, such as sharp drop-offs, must be clearly marked.

❑ Fire extinguishers must be available, suited to the activities, checked regularly, and accessible to all participants.

❑ Adults must know how to use fire extinguishers.

❑ At least one toilet facility and an adjacent hand-washing facility must be provided for every 20 overnight campers.

❑ Garbage disposal plans must be made in advance. If garbage cans are used, they must be insect and animal proof, lined with plastic bags, and kept covered tightly at all times. If no pickup service is available, all garbage must be carried out.

❑ Recycle whenever possible. Buy food and supplies in bulk and avoid excess packaging.

❑ Activities at the site must create an appreciation for the environment with minimal impact.

❏ The site must be left clean (better still, cleaner than it was). "Clean" means removal of trash and evidence of human activities. It does not mean removal of natural materials, such as leaves, from trails.

Primitive campsites (in addition to all points above) must have the following features:

❏ The site must be well below the treeline and away from streams and streambeds, animal dens, partially fallen trees, rock ledges, and potential water runoffs from rain.

❏ Washing areas and latrines must be situated 200 feet away and downhill from any water source.

❏ When there are no established latrines, human waste must be placed in a "cat hole" at least 200 feet away from any water source. The cat hole must be covered after use.

❏ Garbage must be made as compact as possible and carried out of the site for proper disposal.

❏ There must be adequate shelter from possible inclement weather.

❏ Precautions must be taken to protect against harmful insects and ticks, animals, and poisonous plants. Campers must be taught to identify and avoid them.

❏ Mosquito netting and insect repellent must be used where needed.

Additional guidelines may be found in the Backpacking interest project in *Cadette and Senior Girl Scout Interest Projects* or by watching *From Backyard to Backcountry—Camping Lightly on the Land*, a GSUSA slide/cassette tape show about minimal-impact camping.

Emergency Procedures

❏ An adult currently trained in first aid must be present.

❏ A first-aid kit must be available.

❏ Methods of communication with sources of emergency care, such as police, hospitals, and fire officials, must be known and arranged in advance.

❏ An ambulance or other vehicle must be available or on call at all times to transport an injured or sick person.

❏ Telephone numbers for all emergency care and council contacts must be posted where appropriate or carried by the adult in charge, and the location of the telephone must be known.

❏ A day-by-day itinerary must be left at home with a contact person. The contact person must be called upon leaving for the trip and upon return.

❏ Evacuation and emergency plans for severe weather must be written, reviewed, and practiced by girls and leaders. The plan must be posted.

❏ Search-and-rescue procedures for missing persons must be written out in advance, reviewed, and practiced by girls and leaders. The procedures must be posted.

❏ Security plans and procedures must be established and posted.

❏ A fire drill must be practiced on the site, particularly from the sleeping area.

Tubing

(Also refer to Boating activity checkpoints.)

Planning and Supervision

❏ One adult must have certification in Small Craft Safety, Moving Water module from the American Red Cross, or experience in teaching and/or supervising tubing activities.

❏ All girls' comfort level in the water must be assessed, as described in the Boating activity checkpoints on page 70, in order to go tubing.

❏ A minimum of two qualified adults must supervise any tubing activities.

❏ The experienced leader-to-participant ratio for tubing is 1 to 12.

❏ One adult must be the lead tuber; another adult must be the sweep tuber.

❏ Only one person to a tube.

❏ Tubes that are tied together must be secured very snugly with no slack between the tubes.

❏ The adult leader must know first-hand the hazards and rapids on any river to be tubed. All participants must be instructed before beginning to tube.

❏ Girls must receive instruction on how to float through rapids, how to breathe while swimming in rapids, and how to swim to shore.

Clothing

❏ For protection against hypothermia, a wetsuit must be worn when the water temperature is below 65°F.

❏ Laced sneakers or other nonslip footwear designed for water sports must be worn.

Equipment

❏ Each person must wear a PFD.

❏ A container with water or juice must be tied to each tube to allow each girl to replenish fluids.

❏ Use sunscreen and lip balm to prevent sunburn.

Transportation

❏ Transporation arrangements must be made in advance and plans confirmed before departure.

Site

❏ Council guidance must be obtained in selecting a tubing site.

❏ No tubing trip shall be taken on whitewater more difficult than Class II, as defined by the American Version of the International Scale of River Difficulty.

❏ No trip shall be taken on water that has not been run and rated.

❏ The weather report must be known before leaving and monitored during the trip.

Emergency Procedures and First Aid

❏ One adult with current first-aid training must be present.

❏ A first-aid kit must be kept in a waterproof container and secured to a tube.

❏ First-aid procedures must be reviewed, including those for immersion hypothermia, near-drowning, sprains, and fractures.

❏ Arrangements must be made in advance for medical emergencies and evacuation procedures.

Water Skiing

(Also refer to Boating activity checkpoints.)

Planning and Supervision

❏ All instructors must be currently certified by the American Water Ski Association or have equivalent certification or have documented experience, knowledge, and skill in teaching and/or supervising water skiing.

❏ The driver of the boat must be skilled in the operation of the craft, safety and emergency procedures, and management of personnel, and have an appropriate license, if applicable.

❏ The primary certified lifeguard must be an adult.

❏ All water skiing classes must have a minimum of two adults at all times in the boat, one to instruct, lifeguard, and observe the skier(s), and one to drive the boat. The lifeguard must ride in the boat.

❏ Another adult must be on the shore to organize and supervise the girls waiting to ski or watching.

❏ All girls' comfort level in the water must be assessed, as described in the Boating activity checkpoints on page 70, in order to go water skiing.

❏ All persons using the ski boat must be given preliminary training in boarding, debarking, self-rescue in capsizing or swamping situations, boat handling for water skiing, trimming, loading, changing positions, the use of PFDs, and safety procedures for the particular craft.

❏ On a controlled waterfront, a system must be in place for determining the whereabouts of swimmers and boaters, such as a checkboard system.

❏ Ways to signal distress and basic emergency procedures must be understood and practiced.

❏ All participants and instructors must know and practice the hand and voice signals for communication with the ski boat.

❏ The hand and voice signals must be posted at the dock area.

❏ All participants and instructors must know and practice the Water Skier's Safety Code as defined by the American Water Ski Association.

Clothing and Equipment

❏ All participants and instructors must wear a Type III PFD ski vest while on skis or in the ski boat. Ski belts are not acceptable.

❏ Before skiing, proper use of the PFD must be demonstrated and practiced by each person, including an in-the-water experience.

❏ All instructors must have demonstrated knowledge and skill in the operation of the boat, motor, and all specialized skiing equipment.

❏ Ski boats must be seaworthy, fit the water conditions, have sufficient power to tow a skier(s), be appropriate to the skill levels of the participants, and be used only for the purposes designed.

❏ Ski boats must be equipped with a wide-angle rearview mirror.

❏ All federal, state, and locally required equipment for the particular craft and waters must be aboard in serviceable condition, and, if appropriate, labeled "U.S. Coast Guard-approved."

❏ The ski boat must contain at least the following safety equipment:

> ❏ Fire extinguisher
> ❏ First-aid kit
> ❏ Paddle
> ❏ Horn
> ❏ Bailing device
> ❏ Two gas tanks (for outboard motors)
> ❏ Mooring ropes/extra line
> ❏ Boarding ladder
> ❏ Throw bag

❏ All fuel containers must be clearly labeled.

❏ Ski lines (tow lines) must be at least 75 feet in length, in good repair, and of a suitable material.

❑ A single handle must be used on the ski line.

❑ All skis must be appropriate to the skill and size of the skier.

❑ All skis must meet the recommendations as set forth by the American Water Ski Association. Skis must be in good condition.

❑ Skis must be free of sharp points and edges that could cause injury; ski tips must be rounded rather than pointed.

❑ Skis must have properly sized adjustable foot bindings and be the correct length for the skier's weight and planned skiing speed.

Site

❑ Council guidance must be obtained in selecting a water skiing area.

❑ The ski area must meet at least the following description:

> A powerboat moving at 15–25 miles per hour must at least be able to make a straight-line run of a minute or more with a broad sweeping turn at either end. With this "dumb bell" pattern, the boat must be able to remain at least 100 feet from shore at all times (check for state regulations, which may require a greater distance from shore). Thus, the minimum recommended dimensions for a body of water that is closed to other uses during instruction would be approximately 2,000 to 2,400 feet in length and from 250 to 300 feet in width.

❑ There must be a designated pickup and drop-off area for skiers.

❑ The ski dock must be separate from the swimming area and the sailing dock.

❑ Lifeboat and basic rescue equipment must be on hand. Visibility must be good (consider time of day, fog, etc.). Water conditions must be suitable.

❑ Present weather conditions and the long-range forecast must be suitable.

Emergency Procedures and First Aid

❑ An adult with current first-aid training must be present.

❑ The first-aider must be prepared to handle cases of near-drowning and immersion hypothermia.

❑ Arrangements must be made in advance for medical emergencies and severe weather conditions.

National Organization

American Water Ski Association.

Additional activity checkpoints for the following activities can be found in *Safety and Risk Management in Girl Scouting*: Caving, Competitive Orienteering, Kayaking/Touring (Sea), Kayaking (Whitewater), Playgrounds, Ropes Courses and Rappelling, Snowshoeing, and Windsurfing.

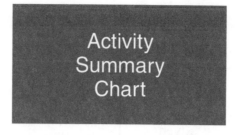

Activity Summary Chart

Safety-Wise requirements for activities (parent/guardian permission is needed for all activities outside the normal troop meeting):

Activity	Council Permission Needed	First-Aider
Archery	yes	yes
Arts and Crafts		
Backpacking	yes	yes
Bicycling	*	yes
Boating	yes	yes
Canoeing	yes	yes
Challenge Courses	yes	yes
Community Activities and Events	yes	yes
Cookie/Council-Sponsored Product Sales	yes	
Cooking, Food Preparation, and Cleaning		
Cooking Fires		yes
Hayrides	*	
Hiking	*	yes
Horseback Riding	yes	yes
Ice Skating	*	yes
Portable Cookstoves		yes
Rafting	yes	yes
Roller Skating	*	yes
Rowboating		yes
Sailing	yes	yes
Science-Related Activities		yes
Skiing (Cross-Country)	*	yes
Skiing (Downhill)	yes	yes
Sports	*	yes
Swimming	*	yes
Theme Park Activities	*	
Trip/Travel Camping	yes	yes
Troop Camping	yes	yes
Tubing	yes	yes
Water Skiing	yes	yes

*Council permission is needed if travel is involved and if the council requires proof of insurance for non-Girl Scout facilities.

Requirements for health histories and health examinations are found in the sections "Program Standards," pages 32–33, and "Basic Safety and Security Guidelines," page 12. See specific activity checkpoints for qualifications of instructors/leaders.

Planning Trips with Girl Scouts

A Girl Scout trip is an opportunity for girls to have fun, to experience adventure, and to enrich ongoing program. Sometimes a trip is the culminating experience in a progression of activities that the girls have already been involved in.

The Planning Process

Learning how to plan a trip should be a progressive experience for a Girl Scout, one that starts with an outing she is ready to handle. Daisy Girl Scouts, for example, might begin with a discovery hike. Even older girls should start with simple trips if they have never done any traveling.

Once the troop, patrol, or other group understands the planning process, girls can progress to longer trips. Whether the trip is a discovery hike or a cross-country trek, the basic steps are essentially the same. The details get more involved as the trip becomes more complex, or when the composition of the group changes, but the process is the same.

Every group that plans a trip starts with the same questions:

Where are we going?

Why are we going?

When are we going?

How will we get there?

How much will it cost?

How should we get ready?

Will everyone be able to go?

Where is emergency help available?

What safety factors must we take into consideration?

What will we do along the way?

What will we do when we get there and when we return home?

The girls answer all the beginning questions in working out their own trip. Through the planning process, they learn how to develop overall plans, make arrangements, budget and handle money, and accept responsibility for personal conduct and safety. Afterward, they evaluate and share the experience with others.

The Progression of Trips

Meeting-Time Trips to points of interest in the neighborhood—for example, a walk to see a nearby garden, or a short ride by car or public transportation to visit a civic building, such as the firehouse or courthouse—are the simplest and start the progression.

Day Trips are the next step. These are day-time excursions away from the troop meeting place and outside the regular meeting time. Girls might plan an all-day visit to a point of historic or natural interest, bringing their own lunches. Or they might go to a nearby city, scheduling time for a meal in a restaurant.

Simple Overnight Trips usually involve one or two nights away. The destination may be a nearby state or national park, a historic site, or a city for sightseeing. The group may stay in a hostel, hotel, or motel; or they may camp out at a Girl Scout campsite or nearby campgrounds.

Extended Overnight Trips can range from three nights or more spent at camp to extensive travel within the continental United States. The group might use several different accommodations and modes of transportation throughout the trip. For further information about travel camping facilities at Girl Scout sites across the country, Girl Scouts of the U.S.A. compiles a Trekking Network Directory, which can be obtained from your council office.

Wider Opportunities are Girl Scout activities/experiences that take place beyond the troop. They can take place in the neighborhood, council, or state, or on a nationwide or international level. Wider opportunities with nationwide participation are promoted annually in *Wider Ops*, which is sent to girls 12 years of age and older and to their leaders.

International Trips Girls who take overnight trips may eventually progress to trips at a greater distance, such as trips to Canada, Mexico, and England. Because of the special requirements of such trips, including regulations and procedures established by the World Association of Girl Guides and Girl Scouts, trips to other countries are dealt with in a special section beginning on page 146.

Progression by Age Level

Troop members vary in their abilities according to the experiences they have had in family or group travel. However, it is still possible to make some generalizations about trips and travel preparations appropriate to each age level.

Reminder: Leaders must always check with the appropriate persons in their council and obtain permission for trips.

Daisy Girl Scouts

Daisy Girl Scout travel activities include an occasional local field trip (up to a day long) or overnight family camping trip. In the Daisy Girl Scout circle, girls can help to decide about specific places they would like to go. For information about such activities, see *The Guide for Daisy Girl Scout Leaders*.

Brownie Girl Scouts

Brownie Girl Scouts go on discovery trips in the neighborhood or nearby places. The idea for taking a trip may come from the girls, or discussion may be stimulated by a leader or an older Girl Scout. In the Brownie Girl Scout Ring, the girls talk about what they would like to do; the leader helps them narrow down their ideas to those that are within their abilities and budget. The girls can then vote on the trip they want and on alternative plans.

For travel of any distance the leader finds how long the trip will take, checks points of interest to Brownie Girl Scouts, and makes arrangements for places to eat and for rest stops. She sets arrival and departure times, schedules tours, arranges transportation, obtains parents' permission. Troop committee members or older Girl Scouts might help with part of these pretrip plans.

In preparation, the Brownie Girl Scouts and their leader talk about what they will see and do on the trip, what they need to bring with them, how much the trip will cost, and what is expected of them, particularly in regard to courtesy and safety.

After the trip, the girls should have the opportunity to discuss and reflect on their trip. Follow-up activities may include dramatizations, stories, or art activities, such as paintings of what impressed them. They should send thank-you notes to anyone who helped make the trip possible or memorable, and might include a painting or a poem they have written. They make plans for future trips, basing these plans on what they have learned, enjoyed, or need to practice.

Junior Girl Scouts

Junior Girl Scouts should read the sections in the *Junior Girl Scout Handbook* that deal with planning trips and safety procedures.

With adult help, the girls choose the place they want to go. The girls do the planning in patrols or small groups, keeping the purpose of the trip in mind. Their planning should include budgeting, pretrip skills, and tips for personal conduct and safety. The leaders advise the girls as needed and, where necessary, help scale down their ideas into what is possible and fun for girls of this age.

Badge activities suggest trips to all kinds of places in the community, as well as hikes, walks, and campouts. Junior Girl Scouts go on day trips in their own communities and to places of interest nearby. As they become experienced in planning and evaluating their adventures, their plans will include longer trips, with stays in hotels or motels as well as camps.

Cadette Girl Scouts

New adventures appeal to Cadette Girl Scouts. Cadette Girl Scouts are ready for a trip of three days or longer if they have successfully completed overnight trips. For example, they might make trips to a state capital or visit with troops in other parts of the country. Contacts with other troops provide ideas to start girls thinking.

Cadette Girl Scouts can successfully combine camp living with exploration and travel, using a campsite as a departure point from which to take trips. Girls with specialized skills—such as riding, biking, skiing, backpacking, or boating—may plan trips around those interests. Girls may also use these skills and interests to prepare for a national wider opportunity, which would provide experiences beyond the troop.

Cadette Girl Scouts can share the excitement of their trip by making exhibits, showing slides, and illustrating log books for their families and friends and for community groups. After several trips, they can share their travel know-how with troops that have less experience. Additional Cadette and Senior Girl Scout travel opportunities are available through the Cadette/Senior Girl Scout Trekking Opportunities listing published by GSUSA, which can be obtained by contacting the local council office.

Senior Girl Scouts

Senior Girl Scout troops and patrols can plan a variety of trips related to their major interests. Because Senior Girl Scouts usually have greater emotional, physical, and mental maturity than younger girls, they have the potential to benefit from more extensive travel. Mature girls, experienced in travel or in the steps of planning, can work with less experienced girls or younger troops. They can help with the planning process, teach specific skills needed for a trip, or serve in a leadership role. They may also use the information in this chapter to prepare for a national or international wider opportunity.

Travel Tips for All Trips

The trip must meet all appropriate program standards listed in the chapter "Girl Scout Program Standards." Particular attention should be given to the appropriate girl/adult ratios for the different age levels.

The adults should learn and share with the troop ahead of time how to access the emergency medical system during trips. Emergency plans should be clearly made prior to departure.

All trip participants should be briefed on the following before a trip:

- What to do if accidentally separated from the group
- What to do if emergency help is needed
- How to deal with the public in a tourist area
- How to perform basic first-aid procedures
- General lifesaving techniques and expected behaviors

Find out in advance about the places to be visited:

- How long it will take to get there and the best means of transportation
- The availability of drinking water, restrooms, and eating places
- Visiting hours and whether advance reservations are needed
- Any physical barriers that cannot be accommodated

Allow enough time for eating, resting, and personal needs while traveling, and have alternative plans in case of bad weather or emergency. When a large group plans to eat in a restaurant, make a reservation and, to save time, consider either ordering meals in advance or ordering the same menu for all. Arrive on time or notify the restaurant if the group will be delayed. Ask about the inclusion of gratuities when a large group is served.

Be sure each girl knows which adult

or patrol leader she is responsible to while on the trip—and that each adult knows the names of the girls she is responsible for. Arrange for an adult contact back home who will be available by phone during the time of the trip. Let that person know of any delay or emergency on the way.

Use the buddy system when traveling. As part of the preparation for any trip, discuss consideration for drivers and other passengers. Wherever possible, arrange in advance for assigned seats in buses, trains, planes, or cars to ensure that every passenger has a seat. On longer trips, rotate seating periodically so that everyone gets a chance at the window seats. Remember to practice emergency evacuation procedures from vehicles.

When making reservations for overnight stops, find out if there is a procedure for preregistering a large group. If there is, one person can check in for the entire group while the others remain in the bus or cars until accommodations are assigned.

Remember, it is not necessary to do everything as a troop while traveling. Provision should be made for breaking into small groups that can pursue special interests in depth during the trip or just have some unscheduled time to relax.

Checklist for Travel Readiness

Here is a checklist of general indicators for leaders and girls to look for in determining whether the troop is ready for a trip. In addition to the travelers themselves, troop consultants and others who help leaders review travel plans should find the checklist useful. Program services personnel can also use the list as they approve travel plans prepared by girls, evaluate trips, and make recommendations relating to trips.

Readiness is shown when the following statements can be made regarding the troop and its plans:

1 The trip is in keeping with Girl Scout policies and standards.

▪ The trip meets all the appropriate program standards listed in the chapter "Girl Scout Program Standards."

2 There is communication with the council.

▪ All appropriate permissions have been obtained from the council.

▪ Leaders and girls know and follow council policies concerning camps and overnight trips, including procedures for handling emergencies.

▪ Council staff are informed of any changes in plans.

3 There is sound planning.

▪ The trip has a clear purpose, formulated and understood by the girls and adults.

▪ The trip is part of ongoing troop activities, with all participants included in the planning steps.

▪ Girls are able to work successfully in groups and are mature enough to accept the responsibilities involved in the trip.

■ The proper number of adult chaperones who are willing to accept the responsibilities of the trip have been recruited.

■ Girls and their parents/guardians are wholeheartedly behind the project; parents/guardians understand all the plans and have confidence in the leadership.

■ All the girls and adults make realistic, detailed plans together well in advance.

■ Plans take into consideration the special abilities and religious and ethnic diversity of the participants, and those of the people with whom they will interact during the trip.

■ Girls and adults learn as much as possible about what they will be seeing and doing.

■ The troop seeks guidance and approval from the council on the kind of transportation that is best for the trip.

4   Travel arrangements are made in advance.

■ Time is provided for eating, sleeping, rest and relaxation, recreation, and personal needs.

■ Mileage to be covered per day is reasonable for the type of terrain expected.

■ Drivers as well as passengers are considered in making plans.

■ Reservations for overnight accommodations are confirmed in writing, and all stopping places are planned in advance.

■ The entire itinerary is known to girls, adults, parents, the council,

and the back-home emergency contact.

5   The business and money matters are worked out.

■ Girls and adults set up a detailed, realistic budget. Remember items such as transportation, food, tips, insurance, recreation, admission fees, taxes, and emergency funds.

■ Money-earning projects are carried on with the permission of the council and in accordance with Girl Scout policies and standards.

■ Personal and group expenses are defined in advance. The amount of personal money that may be needed, and the way those funds should be handled, are determined in advance.

■ Troop travel funds are kept in a bank before the trip, and carried in traveler's checks during the trip.

■ One person is responsible for all troop funds and will keep a daily account of expenditures. However, be sure that not all the cash and traveler's checks are held by just one person at any one time when traveling.

■ Decisions are made in advance concerning how to pay bills that come up prior to the trip, en route, and afterward.

■ For overseas trips, most hospitals and doctors will require cash or credit card payments. Obtain hospital and doctors' bills in English to expedite processing of claims with the insurance company after returning home.

6 Members take responsibility for personal conduct and equipment.

■All girls and adults know what clothing and equipment to take, and how to use and pack the equipment.

■When a troop or group is traveling in the Girl Scout uniform, provision should be made to ensure that all travelers have a uniform. The uniform should be worn correctly. Girls and adults are encouraged to wear the uniform at national centers and to other Girl Guide/Girl Scout activities or events.

■Girls understand their responsibilities as travelers. Everyone is briefed on appropriate conduct and safety precautions in public places, restrooms, building stairs, escalators, elevators, and the selected forms of transportation.

■Groups staying in hotels are prepared to take special precautions to protect their own safety, and also know what to do in case of fire (see "Hotel Security and Safety Tips" in the Appendix, pages 147–148).

■All girls and adults are prepared for new experiences and are open to appreciation of local customs and foods. Local customs and behaviors are explored in advance when traveling internationally.

■On trips requiring special equipment, such as tents, bicycles, canoes, etc., the equipment is checked and ready well before the departure date.

■Luggage and equipment are kept to a minimum. All valuables should be left at home. Individual limits are set and adhered to. Each person is able to carry her own individually identified belongings except when a special consideration, such as a disability, warrants alternative plans.

7 Everyone knows and observes good health and safety practices.

■*Safety-Wise* is used when preparing for any trip. Girls and adults also consult handbooks and leaders' guides for additional information.

■Required health examinations and immunizations are completed. Health records, medical waivers, necessary medications, eyeglass lens prescriptions, and/or extra glasses, are taken along.

■Everyone is physically and mentally able to undertake the trip.

■For trips of a day or more in length, at least one currently trained first-aider is present. Contact the council office to determine which level of first-aid training is needed. Provisions for first aid are made.

■For trips of three nights or more in length, insurance coverage for the entire trip should be obtained through the council under one of the optional accident or accident and sickness plans available.

■Arrangements have been made for an adult contact back home for routine reporting as well as for emergencies.

■Written itineraries, including phone numbers and addresses, are prepared for girls, their families, the council office, and the back-home contact. On overseas trips, the written itineraries include U.S. embassy and consulate locations.

■Procedures for handling accidents, illnesses, and emergencies are understood by all.

■Trip leaders for specialized trips, such as canoeing or backpacking, have taken leadership training related to the activity and are familiar with Girl Scout program standards set forth in *Safety-Wise*. Necessary insurance forms are carried, along with all important papers.

Travel Tips for Girls Traveling Alone

For Cadette and Senior Girl Scouts traveling alone to and from a wider opportunity, special procedures should be designed. These procedures should help the girl feel comfortable and capable of traveling on her own, and should include:

■Assessment of the girl's maturity and ability to handle herself alone by the wider opportunity task group guiding girls through the application, acceptance, and trip-planning process. The assessment should include consultation with the girl's parents or guardians.

■Orientation on hotel and airport security and safety tips. (See pages 147–148.)

■Provision of emergency forms, with telephone numbers of people whom the girl can contact during an emergency if her family is not available, and arrangements for acceptance of emergency collect calls by those listed on the form. Note that the wider opportunity sponsor provides emergency numbers of contact persons at the event site or the arrival point.

■Advice to the girl and her family to book direct flights to and from the event whenever possible, and advice to have the travel agent alert the airline and airport personnel that she is traveling alone. Airlines provide extra help and support for minors traveling alone.

The council can provide the leader and girl with additional information and advice to help ensure a safe trip.

Council-Sponsored Trips

Some councils arrange trips that are open to individual girls, just as they provide other wider opportunities, such as camping, conferences, and volunteer service and Leader-in-Training projects. In sponsoring these trips, the council provides opportunities for girls to pursue special interests if they are willing to devote time for preparation.

Transportation and Travel

Making decisions about transportation is a very important part of planning a trip. The first concern is always safety. But even with the greatest care, when no one is to blame, accidents can happen. Councils have a responsibility to understand the requirements of safety, to evaluate and make recommendations on the kinds of transportation troops/groups use, and then to determine what is best for the trip.

When any trip is being planned, it is important for leaders and girls to work closely with the council from the beginning. Girl Scout leaders do not have the authority to sign agreements or contracts for the rental or charter of vehicles, vessels, and aircraft. This is also the case when the form of transportation is being used without cost. There must be a written agreement even when there is no cost. All contracts and agreements must be submitted to the council to be signed by the person designated by the council board of directors.

Councils must have policies and procedures related to transportation for group travel. Adults and girls who are planning a trip must check with the council before proceeding to be sure that accepted practices are followed. They must follow council guidelines to make certain that both travelers and the council are properly protected by liability insurance in the event of an accident. General liability and automobile liability policies provide insurance for claims or lawsuits arising out of an accident that occurs during a Girl Scout activity.

Choosing Transportation

When selecting any mode of transportation, make certain that the owner/operator is properly licensed, registered, and insured for liability, and that the vehicle is well maintained.

Public Transportation

Transportation companies that commonly serve the public are called common carriers. These are trains and railroads, commercial airlines, bus lines, and ship lines. Common carriers are usually preferable to charters, as they are subject to regulations that set standards for equipment, personnel, and insurance.

Any activity involving chartering, whether aircraft, land vehicle, or watercraft, needs the attention of legal counsel familiar with the appropriate laws. This kind of activity should not be assumed by inexperienced individuals.

Buses

To reach a location that is beyond scheduled routes, the group may want to charter a bus. Under the agreement, the company supplies the vehicle and the driver. The council must be involved in the selection and approval of bus companies.

Council volunteers and staff are not expected to be able to tell if a vehicle is in safe operating order, but they are responsible for checking that vehicles have current registration, that state-mandated safety inspections have been passed, and that obvious defects, such as bald tires, missing or broken lights, cracked or broken glass (including mirrors and windshields), are not present. Contracts with vehicle owners should stipulate that it is the responsibility of the owner to provide a vehicle in safe operating condition and to replace the vehicle or driver if problems develop.

All vehicles traveling on public roads should be equipped with first-aid kits, emergency light/warning reflectors, and fire extinguishers. It is also recommended that vehicles transporting girls be equipped with communication devices such as radio phones or cellular phones whenever possible. The phone numbers for appropriate contacts should be readily available.

The council should have current certificates of insurance on file. When buses are leased or rented with insurance, the council should check with their own insurance agent to determine the minimum amount of insurance that is required by local or state statutes.

When chartering, renting, or borrowing any bus, the following should be considered and verified documentation requested, as appropriate.

- Liability and collision/comprehensive insurance for the vehicle

- Workers' compensation insurance for the driver

- Qualifications, training, and licensing of the driver
- Relief-driver availability
- Familiarity of driver with vehicle
- Sufficient seating and adequate storage space for luggage
- Appropriate emergency equipment

Most states dictate the minimum amount of liability insurance that a vehicle must have. However, some states require none, and the council must judge whether the state minimum is reasonable for the Girl Scout event. The council must also be aware of requirements in other states through which the vehicle will pass. The leader will need to contact the council to find out the amount of liability insurance needed.

Most charter agreements include the provision of a driver.

Some insurance carriers provide insurance only when the owner/operator is using the bus for the owner's purposes—for example, when the school district is using the bus for school district activities. The council needs to be sure that the insurance for the bus will be valid if used for Girl Scout purposes, whether or not the Girl Scouts pay for the use of the bus.

It is the responsibility of the council to furnish a list of transportation providers that can be used when planning Girl Scout activities. Councils should use local or state regulatory authorities to help in determining reputable transportation providers.

Private Passenger Vehicles

Cars, vans, and station wagons are all suitable vehicles for transportation—provided each passenger has a proper seat and seat belt, the vehicle is not overcrowded, and there is adequate insurance.

Every state has motor vehicle laws regulating the licensing of drivers and the registration of vehicles. Most states even dictate the minimum amount of liability insurance required. The leader should contact the council to find out the amount of liability insurance required for the Girl Scout event/activity being planned.

In the event of an accident, the insurance carried by the owner of the vehicle is the primary applicable insurance.

Leased or Rented Vehicles

Read all rental agreements carefully in order to comply with their terms and avoid surprises. Note especially the type and amount of the insurance carried by the rental agency. Rental agreements often specify the minimum age of the driver, from 21 to 25. Know who is responsible for damage to or loss of the vehicle itself. State laws vary greatly on what rental agencies can sell to and/or require of renters in this area. Check with the council to ensure that its nonowned automobile coverage will be effective if needed.

Special Vehicles

Commercial Vehicles, such as flatbed or panel trucks without seats, must never be used to carry passengers. These are utility vehicles designed to transport property. Vehicles such as reconditioned buses that are handmade or cannot be registered as vehicles should not be used to transport passengers. Only vehicles designed to carry passengers can be used to transport

Girl Scouts. Drivers of vehicles with a capacity for more than 15 passengers must have a commerical driver's license.

Recreational Vehicles. When using special vehicles, such as snowmobiles and the like, the following should be considered:

- The owner's liability insurance should be appropriate.
- The vehicle must be maintained in accordance with manufacturer's specifications.
- The vehicle should be driven by an experienced operator over tracks that are free of such obstacles as rocks, fences, barbed wire, and low-hanging branches.
- The vehicle must be registered and/or inspected in compliance with the law.

Campers. Passengers must be transported in seats designed by the manufacturer for that purpose, and seat belts must be worn. Transporting people any other way is dangerous, and may void insurance coverage. Stowage of cargo must be such that sudden stops or impact is not likely to result in damage to passengers. People should not be transported in five-wheel camper/trailers, in campers that fit onto pickup flatbeds, or in the body of any trailer that does not have direct access to the driver.

Air Transportation

Regularly Scheduled Airlines are recommended for Girl Scout group travel. These air carriers provide many choices that have varying costs. Before coming to any decisions, discuss with a travel agent the differences in cost based upon advance booking and off-season and group fares.

Private Planes. The poor accident records of private planes, especially those owned by companies, is the primary reason this form of transportation is discouraged. Other factors involve the inability of a Girl Scout council to evaluate the pilot's qualifications and the mechanical condition of the plane. A private plane owner is not required to meet the same federal standards applicable to commercial aircraft. Flying in small private planes is not permitted as a Girl Scout program activity.

Charter Flights. Chartering of planes by Girl Scout troops involves legal and financial responsibilities, and additional, specialized liability insurance must be purchased. Any agreements to charter flights must be approved and signed by the council. Generally, the chartering of planes is not recommended, as it is impractical for Girl Scout councils.

Watercraft Transportation

In recent years the regulation of boating by both the federal and state governments has been increasing. The council must be sure that craft used meet the standards of the regulatory agency having authority in the jurisdiction.

The chartering of boats longer than 16 feet, with or without a crew, is not recommended. Special licenses for certain crew members are usually required, and Admiralty Law makes the charterer usually responsible not only for any damage

to the boat, but often damage to other boats and the pollution of waterways, and may even require the removal of sunken vessels from navigable waters.

All vessels carrying passengers must be registered or documented according to federal regulations and state statute. They are also inspected according to U.S. Coast Guard or state regulation (depending on number of passengers, size of vessel, means of propulsion, and water routes). PFDs (life jackets) are easily accessible and available in an appropriate size for each passenger. Operators of vessels carrying passengers are licensed as required by federal regulations or state statute.

Vessels must not be overloaded. The number of persons aboard must not exceed the recommended or certified capacity. Luggage and equipment must be stowed securely and in a way that will help keep the vessel stable.

The securing of adequate liability insurance for chartered passenger-carrying vessels should be thoroughly investigated prior to entering any charter arrangements.

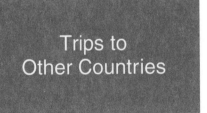

Trips to
Other Countries

As noted on page 127, girls who take overnight trips may eventually progress to trips outside the country. Trips to Canada or Mexico are a good introduction to international travel and a chance for girls to practice being good ambassadors. Trips across the ocean require two or three years of preparation and are undertaken by relatively few troops or council-sponsored groups.

Before initiating trips to other countries, including Canada and Mexico, the group and the adults in charge should have demonstrated to the council their ability to plan, organize, budget, accept responsibility, observe emergency and safety measures, work together as a group, and evaluate their experiences through a variety of successful short and extended trips.

As soon as there is interest in traveling outside the country, leaders and girls should inform the council and get permission to plan the trip. They should work with the council from the beginning and establish a timetable and checkpoints for reporting progress as plans develop. Be sure to secure final council permission and other permissions as required along the way.

Preparation Packet

A preparation packet for Girl Scout groups planning an international trip is available from your local Girl Scout council. This packet contains information about immunizations and other health precautions for international travelers; working with a travel agent; obtaining passports and other needed documents; learning about other countries and cultures; financing an international trip; what to take and how to pack; resources on Girl Scouting and Girl Guid-

ing around the world; and general advice on how to make your travel dreams come true.

Several sections include helpful hints—"Things I wish I'd known"— from girls who have actually traveled abroad. All Girl Scout groups that are planning trips to other countries are advised to obtain this packet.

Do not contact Girl Guide/Girl Scout association offices in other countries for information or for help with travel plans. Most of the Girl Guide/Girl Scout offices around the world are very small and are staffed by only a handful of people. To ensure that these people are not overwhelmed with correspondence, all communication between Girl Guide/Girl Scout organizations is carried on only by the international commissioners. GSUSA's international commissioner can be contacted by writing to International Commissioner, c/o National/International Relations, GSUSA, 420 Fifth Avenue, New York, N.Y. 10018-2702.

Travel Procedures for Visiting the Juliette Gordon Low Girl Scout National Center

The Juliette Gordon Low Girl Scout National Center provides year-round program opportunities for troops and groups. For troops and groups planning to visit the Birthplace, reservations must be made in advance. Families and individuals do not need a reservation for a tour. Write directly to the Juliette Low center at 142 Bull Street, Savannah, Georgia 31401, or call (912) 233-4501 to request a copy of *Birthplace Bound*, a detailed booklet about sessions, rates, lodging, camping, restaurants, and sightseeing.

Travel Procedures for Visiting WAGGGS Centers or Member Countries

For groups that want to stay at a world center or Girl Guide hostel, or simply want to visit the Girl Guide/Girl Scout headquarters in countries where there is a WAGGGS organization, specific procedures must be followed.

Procedures for travel to Canada are included in the Appendix (page 144), along with an application form. The procedures and form may be reproduced by councils as needed.

Intent to Travel Forms A and B are available from the council office along with procedures for their use, and may be reproduced by councils as needed.

■ Intent to Travel Form A is for travelers who plan to stay at a world center or Girl Guide hostel.

■ Intent to Travel Form B is for individuals or groups who plan to visit a world center or a member country of the World Association of Girl Guides and Girl Scouts while they are traveling abroad and wish to obtain a Card of Introduction.

The Card of Introduction is recognized by all Girl Guide and Girl Scout associations throughout the world as the standard form of introduction. Through GSUSA's membership in the World Association, the card is available to Girl Scouts to facilitate contact with Girl Guides in the countries to be visited. The card does not, however, entitle travelers to request hospitality or services. Requests of this nature are inappropriate and should not be made.

Timetable

One to two years before the trip, the leader planning to visit or stay at a world center or Girl Guide hostel completes Intent to Travel Form A and sends it to the council. The council sends a copy to the Program Group at GSUSA, provides guidance for the troop or group, and reminds the leader to confirm dates, itinerary, and the list of girl and adult travelers six to eight weeks before departure. The Program Group responds to the leader, sending the information requested on the Intent to Travel form.

Six to eight weeks before the trip, the leader confirms to the council dates, itinerary, insurance coverage, and list of travelers. The council sends the endorsed Intent to Travel Form B to the Program Group at GSUSA. Cards of Introduction are sent to the leader. Travelers requesting Cards of Introduction less than a month in advance cannot be assured of receiving them before departure.

Individuals may follow the same procedures, notifying the council of travel plans in advance if planning to visit or stay at a world center or Girl Guide hostel. Or, if they need only Cards of Introduction, individual travelers may inform the council six to eight weeks in advance of their plans, travel dates, itinerary, and names of travelers. The council sends an endorsed copy of Intent to Travel Form B to the Program Group. A Card of Introduction is sent to the individual.

After Any Trip

When any trip is over, all bills should be paid promptly. Girls and adults should write thank-you letters to people who helped along the way and return borrowed or rented equipment in good condition.

Evaluate the trip. Discuss what was fun and worthwhile, decide what girls and adults would like to change or eliminate on future trips, and report back to the council with the troop's evaluation.

Find ways for the troop to build new activities based on their travel experiences. Share the experiences with others and don't forget the people in the community who helped with the group's preparations. The group will also want to pass tips along to other Girl Scouts who are planning similar trips.

Encourage girls to keep in touch with friends made along the way. Someday these friends might be travelers visiting your area.

Traveling in Cyberspace

Using computers to travel through cyberspace can be fun, but as with any trip, girls should be prepared for unforeseen things. If girls are working on technology projects or recognitions, provide each of them with a copy of this pledge. Ask each to discuss it with a parent or adult partner who is doing computer activities with her.

My Online Safety Pledge

■ I will not give out personal information such as my address, telephone number, work address/telephone number of my parents/guardian, or the name and location of my school without the permission of my parents/guardian.

■ I will tell an adult right away if I come across any information that makes me feel uncomfortable.

■ I will never agree to get together with someone I "meet" online without first checking with my parents/guardian. If my parents/guardian agree to the meeting, I will be sure that it is in a public place and bring a parent/guardian along.

■ I will never send a person my picture or anything else without first checking with my parents/guardian.

■ I will not respond to any messages that are mean or in any way make me feel uncomfortable. It is not my fault if I get a message like that. If I do, I will tell my parents/guardian right away so that they can contact the online service.

■ I will talk with my parents/guardians so that we can set up rules for going online. We will decide upon the time of day that I can be online, the length of time I can be online, and appropriate areas for me to visit. I will not access other areas or break these rules without their permission.

Girl Scout _____ Date _____

Adult Partner _____ Date _____

Appendix

Sample Parent Permission Form

Troop/Group _____ is planning a _____

Date _____ Time _____

Location _____ Phone number _____

Arrangements for transportation:

Time and place of departure _____

Time and place of return _____

Mode of transportation _____

Leaders accompanying the girls:

Name(s) _____

_____

Each girl will need:

Expenses _____

Equipment and clothing _____

_____

_____

In case of an emergency, the leader will notify:

Name _____ Phone number _____

    who will immediately notify the parents.

_____   _____

Leader's signature   Phone number

Return this page to troop leader

My daughter _____

has permission to participate in _____

   She can participate with reasonable accommodations.   Yes _____   No _____

   Please describe. _____

   _____

   _____

   During the activity, I may be reached at:

   Address _____

   _____ Phone number _____

   If I (we) cannot be reached in the event
   of an emergency, the following person is
   authorized to act in my (our) behalf:

   Name and address _____

   _____

   _____

   Relationship to participant _____ Phone number _____

   Physician's name _____ Phone number _____

   Additional remarks: _____

   _____

   _____

   _____

   _____

   _____

   _____

   _____

   _____

_____
Parent or guardian's signature

_____
Date

Sample Letter to a Program Consultant

Dear Consultant:

We are pleased that you have accepted an opportunity to work with the Girl Scouts as a consultant. Your services are being requested because you have a special interest (expertise, hobby, or skill) that you can share with girls.

Girl Scouts have much to gain from meeting and working with adults from the community. Every girl with whom you work may not become an expert in your field of special interest. However, through your help, each girl can increase her awareness and knowledge of the world and gain full useful skills. Girls can discover worthwhile leisure activities as well as new career directions.

Girl Scouting is a movement that gives girls from all segments of American life a chance to develop their potential, to make friends, and to become a vital part of their community. Based on ethical values, it opens up a world of opportunity for youth working in partnership with adult volunteers.

Its program is a continuous adventure in learning that offers girls a broad range of activities that address both their current interests and their future roles as women. Through activities that stimulate self-discovery, girls are introduced to the excitement in the worlds of science, the arts, the out-of-doors, and people. Girls grow in skill and in self-confidence. They have fun, they make friends, and through meaningful community service they acquire understanding about themselves and others. During these activities the protection and safety of girls are paramount.

We hope that you will be able to enrich the Girl Scout experience for (*describe girls who will benefit—age levels, number, etc.*) by (*describe requested service of consultant*).

We are of the (*name of council*) Council. I look forward to discussing more with you in the near future.

Sincerely yours,

Procedures for Camping and Other Across-the-Border Visits of More Than 48 Hours in Canada

Girl Scouts of the U.S.A. and Canada have cooperatively established procedures for camping and across-the-border visits of more than 48 hours. To maintain the goodwill fostered by these exchanges, complete the application and follow these procedures.

The leader, at least three months in advance of the proposed trip, notifies the council that the group is planning a trip to Canada and wishes to visit and/or camp with Canadian Girl Scouts.

The council gives the leader an application form (three copies).

The leader completes the form, keeps one copy, and returns the other two to the council for approval.

The council, if it approves the trip, keeps one form and forwards one copy of the form to the appropriate Canadian Provincial International Commission requesting clearance.

The Canadian Provincial International Commissioner, after negotiation with her areas, writes directly to the leader indicating what, if any, part of the request can be met, and the name and address of the person in Canada with whom the leader can correspond and plan. A copy of this letter is sent to the council.

From this point on, the negotiations proceed between the leader and her Canadian contact.

The U.S.A. Girl Scout troop leader must be sure she has:

- Clear directions for the destination of the group (camp, city, home, office, etc.).

- The name and phone number of the person in Canada to be contacted in case plans must be changed, or in case the group cannot find its destination. (If the phone number of the destination is different from the phone number of the contact person, leaders should have this number as well.)

Additional Information

It is not possible to arrange for camping at Girl Guide campsites or contact with Canadian Guides for visits shorter than 48 hours.

Girl Scout troops and their leaders should realize that there may be times when the numbers of Girl Scouts requesting camping privileges and Guide contacts make it impossible for the Canadian Girl Guides to fulfill every request.

Canadian contacts should not be expected to provide tourist information. This may be obtained by writing the Department of Tourism in the capital of the province where you will be traveling. There are also Canadian government travel bureaus in some of the major U.S. cities.

Girl Guides of Canada will follow similar procedures for across-the-border visits and camping in the U.S.A.

Girl Scouts of the U.S.A./Girl Guides of Canada Application for Camping and Other Across-the-Border Visits of More Than 48 Hours

Council name _____

Council address _____
Street

_____
City   State   Zip

Troop leader's name _____ Troop No. _____

Address _____
Street

_____
City   State   Zip

Trip Plans

Approximate number of girls _____ between the ages of _____ and _____

Approximate number of adults _____

Will be traveling by _____
(Plane, train, public bus, chartered bus, private cars)

We plan to stay the following nights: (attach extra sheets if necessary)

	Date	City	Province	Reservation made: name and address of hotel/motel/camp
1st Day	_____	_____	_____	_____
2nd Day	_____	_____	_____	_____
3rd Day	_____	_____	_____	_____

We would like Girl Guides to join us for (check): daytime activities on _____ ; evening campfire on _____ ; overnight stay on _____ ; and/or we would like to join with Girl Guides if they are having any event on the following dates _____ .

We would like to camp on a Canadian Guide campsite in the vicinity of

_____ from _____ to _____
(city and province)

with a group of Girl Guides _____ (yes) _____ (not necessarily).

The following person will know where our troop is during each day of our trip and is the person who should be contacted in case of emergency:

Name _____ Telephone number _____
Area code

Address _____

_____
Troop leader's signature

_____
Signature of council representative giving approval for trip   Date

Leaders of groups wishing to stay at a world center or Girl Guide hostel or wishing to obtain a World Association Card of Introduction must follow the procedures listed below.

Stay at a World Center or Girl Guide Hostel

1 **One to two years before departure,** obtain "Intent to Travel Form A: Request for International Travel Materials" from your Girl Scout council. Complete and send to:

Membership and Program Services
Girl Scouts of the U.S.A.
420 Fifth Avenue
New York, New York 10018–2798

You will receive an Accommodations Request Form and materials containing information about the world center(s) you specify. For an international preparation packet, contact your council.

2 **Six months to two years before departure,** as indicated on the form or in the accompanying materials, send the Accommodations Request Form and necessary International Reply Coupons (obtainable from U.S. Post Offices) to the center or hostel.

3 **Upon receipt of confirmation of reservations,** send registration fees in the currency requested to the center or hostel.

4 **Six to eight weeks before departure,** send arrival confirmation (from Accommodations Request Form) to the center or hostel.

Send "Intent to Travel Form B: Request for World Association Card of Introduction" to the council for endorsement and then to Membership and Program Services, GSUSA.

Visit the Headquarters of a WAGGGS Association

Six to eight weeks before departure, send "Intent to Travel Form B: Request for World Association Card of Introduction" to Membership and Program Services, GSUSA.

A card will not be issued more than three months in advance of departure. Travelers requesting cards of introduction less than one month in advance cannot be assured of receiving them prior to departure.

Hotel Security and Safety Tips

While every reputable hotel works hard to ensure the safety and security of its guests, the cooperation and safety consciousness of each individual guest are still essential. For that reason, leaders of Girl Scout groups that will be staying in hotels should make sure that every member of the group is thoroughly familiar with the following safety and security tips.

In the Hotel

When you enter your hotel sleeping room, always lock the door behind you. Use the chain, if there is one.

If there's a knock at your door, ask who it is before you open the door. Don't hesitate to call the desk to confirm that a hotel staff person is at your door.

Don't call your room number out to a friend while in the hotel's lobby or hallways. You never know who may be listening.

Don't display your key (with your room number on it) at any time, especially in the elevator on the way to your room.

Valuables

Leave all irreplaceable possessions at home. Do not attempt to hide any item in your hotel room. Use the hotel safety deposit boxes, when available. Do not take valuable jewelry on a trip! If you do, wear it or carry it with you at all times. Never leave jewelry in your hotel room.

Carry your camera with you at all times.

Never leave cash, traveler's checks, personal checks, passports, or credit/charge cards in your hotel room.

Luggage

Never leave luggage unattended at the hotel or airport. As an added precaution, you may want to lock your suitcase when you leave your hotel room. However, most thieves know how to open a locked suitcase.

Lost/Missing Items

If you discover something is missing, notify the hotel's security office or the police or both as quickly as possible. A list of credit card numbers and traveler's check numbers will help.

Fire Safety

Pack a small flashlight to keep on your bedside table with the room key, wallet, and/or passport. A fire can cause failure in the hotel's electrical system.

Read carefully the fire safety information you will find in your hotel room upon arrival. Be sure to:

- Locate the emergency exits on your floor.

- Locate the nearest fire alarm and read the instructions.

If you smoke, be especially careful about smoking in your hotel room. Smoldering cigarettes are a major cause of hotel fires. It is expected that girls will not be smoking.

Select a specific place, such as the bedside table, where you will put your room key while in your hotel room. This will enable you to locate the key quickly in case of an emergency.

In case of fire, follow the instructions in the hotel's fire safety information.

If there's a fire alarm or warning call from the hotel management, get out as quickly as possible. Don't stop to gather personal belongings. Do take your room key, flashlight, and wallet/passport, as you may find it necessary to go back to your room. Without a key you may be locked out of your room, which may be a safer place to be if the hallways or stairwells are dense with smoke.

Before leaving the room, feel the door to the corridor. If the door is warm, do not open it. If the door is cool, open it slowly with your foot or shoulder propped against it so you can slam it shut if heavy smoke or flames are visible.

If the hallway looks safe, go to the nearest emergency exit. If there is smoke in the corridor, put a wet towel over your face to reduce smoke inhalation and stay low. Close all doors behind you to help block the fire's spread.

When you reach the emergency exit, again feel the door. If it's hot, then the fire is in that stairwell, so use an alternate exit.

Never use the elevators during a fire unless instructed or accompanied by the fire department. Many elevator controls are heat sensitive and will take you to the floor where the fire is located.

If your hotel room door is warm or the hallway is dense with smoke, stay in your room and seal spaces around the door with wet towels. Call the hotel operator to report your situation.

Above all, keep a cool head. The byproducts of fire—smoke, poisonous gases, and panic—cause the great majority of fire deaths. Be prepared . . . and be a survivor.

Lifesaving Awards

Lifesaving awards have been part of Girl Scout program since the beginning of the Movement in the United States. Lifesaving awards are a form of recognition given to a registered Girl Scout (not an adult) who has saved or attempted to save human life under circumstances that indicate heroism or risk of her own life. They are reserved for those Girl Scouts who have performed heroic acts beyond the degree of maturity and training to be expected at their age.

A Girl Scout, in accordance with the Girl Scout Promise and Law, motto, and slogan to which she has subscribed, is expected to be resourceful, skilled, and competent—to have presence of mind and to be of service to others. Determining whether an act constitutes unusual bravery and is beyond what is generally expected of a Girl Scout is often difficult. Each situation has unique factors, and many things need to be taken into consideration—for example, degree of difficulty of the rescue, amount of assistance received from others, and the circumstances surrounding the incident. If a leader determines that the action of a Girl Scout may merit a lifesaving award, she should contact her Girl Scout council to obtain information about the awards and application procedures.

The judgment on the merit of an act that could qualify for a lifesaving award is a responsibility of the local council. The council, being close to the specific situation, is in a position to gather the facts rapidly, check them for accuracy of detail, and use judgment in determining whether an act really merits a lifesaving award.

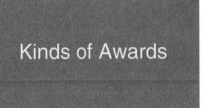

Kinds of Awards

Bronze cross—is given for saving a life or attempting to save a life with risk to the candidate's own life.

Medal of honor—is given for saving a life or attempting to save a life without risk to the candidate's own life.

When a rescue does not qualify for either of these national awards, the council may give the girl some form of local recognition. The type of recognition awarded should be determined by the nature of the rescue.

Glossary

Adult: The age of majority as defined by state statute.

Biodegradable: Anything capable of being decomposed by natural biological processes.

Buddy System: A safety practice in which girls are paired to keep watch over each other. In an activity (for example, swimming, hiking) the girls paired should be of equal ability.

Bungee Jumping: Jumping from a structure, such as a bridge, with a bungee cord attached to the body. This is not a recommended Girl Scout activity.

Cat Hole: A primitive sanitation method used if a toilet or a latrine is not available. It is made by scraping away the upper layer of soil 6–8 inches with the heel or a trowel. Cover the waste with soil and carry out used toilet paper in a plastic bag for proper disposal.

Certified: Holds a current (not expired) card, certificate, or other documentation from an established, reputable group for the level of training required for the activity being conducted.

Chase Boat: See definition under "Lifeboat."

Checkboard System: A swimmer's safety check. Each swimmer has a numbered tag hung on a board. She reverses her tag on the board before going into the water, then turns it over when she returns. The waterfront supervisor can then tell exactly how many persons are swimming at a given moment.

Checkpoint: Quick reference to specific activities.

Community Camping Event: A troop/group camping event organized and operated by volunteers in a geographic subdivision of the council. The community must have approval from the council to operate and must follow the guidelines in *Safety Management at Girl Scout Sites and Facilities*. Each troop is responsible for some of its own plans and scheduling, and also takes advantage of activities planned for the entire group. The site may be council-owned, leased, rented, or borrowed. Usually a two- to three-day event.

Contact Person: The person to get in touch with in case of emergencies or for guidance and advice.

Controlled Waterfront: An area where hazards have been eliminated and the water is known to be free from dangerous marine life, debris, and sharp stones and shells. Diving and boating areas are clearly marked or roped off.

Core Staff: Those persons designated by the council to help girls and leaders carry out their specific troop camping plans at a given campsite (for example, site director, waterfront staff, naturalist, craft specialist).

Counselor-in-Training (CIT): A qualified Senior Girl Scout who is taking a Counselor-in-Training course to learn outdoor group leadership skills.

Day Camping: Camping by the day or camping within a 12-hour program day (this need not be limited to 3 p.m. to 9 p.m., 7:30 a.m. to 3:30 p.m., or 12:30 p.m. to 8:00 p.m.). Girls from different troops sign up as individual campers and are placed in temporary troops (units). The girls and unit staff plan and carry out activities. Day camping is council-sponsored (requires council approval to operate), and the council provides the staff, facilities, and site. The site may be council-owned, leased, rented, or borrowed.

Deadfall: Dry wood, found on the ground, that has fallen off a tree.

Documented Training and Experience: Written evidence of competence in a leadership role. This may include records of previous leadership and/or training to instruct the activity, course completion certificates or cards, letters of reference, and/or written evaluation of previous successful leadership work.

Drugs: Includes all prescription medications as well as all over-the-counter drugs that are potentially hazardous if misused (e.g., aspirin, cold tablets).

Emergency Procedures: Basic plans established in advance stating what should be done in case of emergency. Plans should be established orally as well as in writing, and should be posted in a highly visible location.

EPA: Environmental Protection Agency.

Equivalent Training and/or Certification: Course contents that include all of the elements required by a nationally recognized certifying body at the advanced or instructor level for that skill.

Excursion: A troop/group trip away from a base camp (day or resident) of not longer than one night and two days' duration, planned and carried out by the troop/group and its leader, using motorized transportation, with the destination being a particular point of interest.

Extended Trip: A trip lasting more than three days, thus requiring a health examination in addition to a health history.

Fall Zone: The surface under and around a piece of playground equipment onto which a child falling from or exiting the playground equipment would be expected to land.

First-Aider: An adult who has taken first-aid training as approved by the Girl Scout council. The level of first aid is determined by the nature of the program activity. A first-aider must be currently certified and take refresher training as required by the sponsoring organization. The following may serve as first-aiders at Level 2: physician, physician's assistant, pediatric nurse practitioner, registered nurse, paramedic, military medic, and emergency medical technician.

Float Plan: A detailed itinerary that gives pertinent details for an intended trip in a watercraft. It should include departure and return times, total length of time on water, list of persons on craft, where and when the stops will be made, and the route to be taken.

Frostbite: The freezing of body parts as a result of exposure to extremely low temperatures.

Fund Raising: Techniques to appeal to the public for contributed funds to support the program and activities of the organization. Fund raising often relates to short-term needs and is only part of a fund development plan.

Giardia Lamblia: An organism found in many natural water sources that can cause intestinal discomfort, diarrhea, loss of appetite, and dehydration if ingested.

Girl Scout Camping: An experience that provides a creative, educational opportunity in group living in the out-of-doors. Its purpose is to utilize Girl Scout program, trained leadership, and the resources of natural surroundings to contribute to each camper's mental, physical, social, and spiritual growth.

Head Count: A method of keeping track of the number of participants at a given activity by periodically counting the participants to make sure they are present.

Health Examination: A physical checkup given by a licensed physician, a qualified nurse practitioner, a physician's assistant, or a registered nurse under a physician's orders within the 24 months preceding a girl's participation in resident camping, in a trip of more than three nights, or in contact sports on an organized competitive basis. Health examination forms are available from the Girl Scout council office.

Health History: An annual updated record of the girl's past and present health status (for example, allergies, chronic illnesses, and injuries) that is to be completed by the parent or guardian. A health history is required before a girl participates in physically demanding activities, such as water sports, horseback riding, or skiing. Health history forms are available from Girl Scout council offices.

Heat Exhaustion: The body's reaction of dehydration and prolonged exposure to high temperatures. Symptoms include fatigue, weakness, and collapse. Also called heat prostration.

Heatstroke: A life-threatening condition characterized by extremely high body temperature and disturbance of the sweating mechanism.

"Hot Dog" Skiing: Gymnastic-type skiing consisting of flips and other acrobatics. Because of its unpredictable variables, "hot dog" skiing is not recommended as a Girl Scout program activity.

Hypothermia: A state of lowered internal body temperature—a life-threatening condition.

Itinerary: The planned route to be followed on a journey or trip. (Includes places, dates, and lengths of stay.)

Kindling Point: The temperature at which something will start to burn.

Leader: A registered Girl Scout adult who has received training and who meets regularly with girls to help them achieve the purposes of Girl Scouting.

Leader-in-Training (LIT): A qualified Senior Girl Scout who is taking a Leader-in-Training course to learn leadership skills.

Lifeboat, Chase Boat, or Rescue Boat: A square-sterned boat equipped with oars, oarlocks, life rings, throw bags or other life-saving devices; a stocked first-aid kit that includes a single-use pocket face mask; a personal flotation device; and a motor and fuel container if allowed by regulation.

Lifeguard: A person who holds current certification in the skills and techniques of lifeguarding from a recognized sponsoring agency and has received additional training specific to the facility/body of water where she/he will guard. The lifeguard will have training in first aid and cardiopulmonary resuscitation. The type of certification needed will depend on the type of facility/body of water where the activity takes place.

Minimal-Impact Camping (low-impact camping): Camping in which no trace of activities is left. The physical landscape of the campsite is preserved as well as the solitude and spirit of the wilderness.

Outdoor Day: A special outdoor event, planned and operated by a council or carried out with council permission. Attendance is sometimes by troop, sometimes by individual girl members. The event may involve one to several troops, may be councilwide, or may be intercouncil in scope.

Outdoor Education: The effective utilization of Girl Scout program in the outdoor setting to enable girls to grow with regard to each of the four Girl Scout program goals.

Passengers (on watercraft): Persons other than the operator, the owner and crew, and employees on board a vessel, except guests on board for pleasure who have not contributed any consideration, directly or indirectly, for their carriage. (U.S. Coast Guard definition.)

Passenger Vessel: A vessel carrying passengers (see definition above). When in United States navigable waters, such a vessel is subject to U.S. Coast Guard inspection and licensing regulations.

Patrol: A group of girls no larger than eight, with a girl leader; usually a subdivision of a Girl Scout troop.

Personal Flotation Device (PFD): A life jacket, life preserver, buoyant vest, ring buoy, buoyant cushion, or special-purpose water safety buoyant device designed to keep a person afloat in the water.

Policy: An established course of action that must be followed. The "Policies of Girl Scouts of the United States of America" are found in the *Blue Book of Basic Documents* and in the accompanying *Leader's Digest*.

Portable Cookstove: A stove that uses liquid or canister fuel.

Preschool Age: Children from two years of age to not more than five years of age.

Primitive Camp (or outpost camp): A portion of a permanent or other campsite where the basic needs for camp operation, such as places of abode, water supply systems, and permanent toilet and cooking facilities, are not usually provided.

Product Sales, Council-Sponsored: Councilwide sales of authorized, tangible products, such as Girl Scout cookies or calendars, in which troops may participate.

Program Consultant: A person who shares her or his interests and special abilities with troop members, usually by working directly with girls but sometimes by advising or instructing leaders or camp staff.

Program Emphases: See program goals, pages 30–31.

Qualified Instructor: An instructor who has taken training in the activity to be conducted and has a current certification.

Restricted Water: A water area that has limited space available for steering—for example, docking and mooring areas.

Risk: The possibility of uncertain danger, harm, or loss.

Safe Drinking Water: Water from a tap that has been tested by the local health department. All natural water sources are considered potentially contaminated and should be purified before use. Once water has been purified, it should be stored in a clean, covered container. In areas where *Giardia lamblia* is present, special precautions must be taken. This protozoan is of increasing concern to backcountry campers. If present in the water source, *Giardia* can be removed only by boiling the water or pouring it through specially designed filters. Ingestion of *Giardia* can cause diarrhea, loss of appetite, dehydration, and cramps.

Safety Belay: A means of stopping the descent of a person on a ropes course by means of an additional climbing rope controlled by a trained belayer.

Safety Helmet: A protective headgear with chin strap. Different kinds are made for use while biking, canoeing, and horseback riding and usually have a seal from an approving authority.

Sailing School Vessel: A vessel carrying six or more sailing school students or instructors and operated exclusively for sailing instruction (seamanship, oceanography, maritime history, etc.).

Sensitive Issues: Topics highly personal in nature or rooted in beliefs and values, i.e., AIDS, child abuse, human sexuality, and religion.

Small Craft: Watercraft under 26 feet in length, which may include rowboats, canoes, inflatable boats, and sailing craft.

Standard: An established level of quality or achievement for measuring and judging a council's performance in delivering Girl Scout program to girls.

Swim Test: A test that determines a person's ability to handle herself when pitched into the water.

Topography: The physical or natural features of the landscape. A topographical map details manmade features, bodies of water, vegetation, and elevation of the landscape.

Travel Camping: A travel experience carried out by groups of girls using campsites as a means of accommodation or traveling groups using other than campsites as a means of accommodation, and by adult leadership. Motorized transportation is used to move the group from one site to another over a period of three or more nights. Motorized transportation is normally a van, bus, or automobile; but it may also be an airplane, boat, train, or combination of these vehicles.

Trip Camping: A camping experience planned and carried out by a group of girls who are experienced campers and adult leaders. The group camps at different sites for three or more nights and travels from one site to another under its own power or by transportation that permits individual guidance of the vehicle or animal—for example, bicycle, canoe, horse, or sailboat.

Trip Leader: An adult who accompanies a troop/group on a trip such as camping, backpacking, or canoeing. She/he possesses the knowledge, skills, and experience for the trip being taken. Some of these areas include outdoor leadership, trip planning, risk management, first aid, and supervision.

Troop/Group Camping: A camping experience of 24 or more consecutive hours, planned and carried out by a troop of Girl Scouts and troop leaders, using sites approved by the council. The site may be noncouncil-owned or council-owned, leased, rented, or borrowed.

Troop Money Earning: Any activity planned or carried out by girls and supported by adults, in partnership, to earn money for the troop treasury.

Unit: (1) A small group or troop formed at a day or resident camp; campers are assigned to a unit on the basis of age or interest or both for the entire camp session. (2) That portion of a campsite designated as the living and working area for a troop or unit of campers.

Vehicle: Any device, contrivance, or vessel for carrying or conveying persons or objects.

Vessel: A craft for navigation of water; a watercraft.

Watcher: A person trained in the use of basic water rescue equipment and practices who works under the direction of the lifeguard. American Red Cross Basic Water Rescue certification or equivalent is appropriate.

Whitewater: A froth of water containing air, usually associated with rapid currents in narrow or obstructed channels. Whitewater is not dense enough to float a person. A person can easily drown in whitewater.

Types of whitewater are classified in the International Scale of River Difficulty by the American Whitewater Affiliation. If rapids on a river generally fit one of the following classifications but the water temperature is below 50° F, or if the trip is an extended one into a wilderness area, the river should be considered one class more difficult than normal.

Class I:
Moving water with a few riffles and small waves. Few or no obstructions.

Class II:
Easy rapids with waves up to three feet, and clear channels that are obvious without scouting. Some maneuvering is required.

Class III:
Rapids with high, irregular waves often capable of swamping an open canoe. Narrow passages that often require complex maneuvering. May require scouting from above.

Classes IV, V, VI:
Increasingly turbulent, violent rapids with conditions that make navigability and rescue difficult or impossible. Classes V and VI are unsuitable for canoes.

Index

Program 3/93